GW00707437

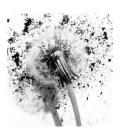

themomentis**now**

For June Frost,
Leader of the
Wednesday Healing Clinic.
With much love and
without whom,
this world would be
so much poorer.

For all my helpers along the way:
the unseen,
the healers,
the College,
themomentisnow and
Chiron and Lily

LOTTERY FUNDED

The Tree of Light
Working creatively with longterm illness

Tina Lawlor Mottram

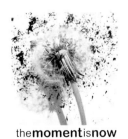

the**moment**isnow

The Tree of Light
Working creatively with longterm illness
Published April 2010

ISBN 978-1-907597-00-8

Published by
The**momentisnow**!
Sunlight Development Trust
105 Richmond Road
Gillingham
Kent ME7 1LX
www.sunlighttrust.org.uk
www.themomentIsnow.org.uk

Email sales
serpentina@blueyonder.co.uk
tinalm@sunlighttrust.org.uk

Printed and bound in Britain by
BigSkyprint.com

Design: Serpentina Creations
www.serpentinacreations.com
Cover Design: James Solly, Doug Fry, Tina Lawlor Mottram

Contents

Max Eames,
President, in
his office at
the College
of Psychic
Studies in
2009.

Below:
1. Pinhole
photograph of
the College.
2. Portrait gallery
on the stairs to
the healing clinic.
3. The library.

*Photographs by
David Wise*

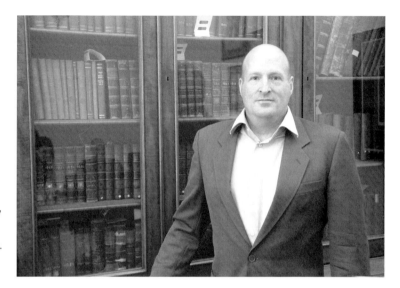

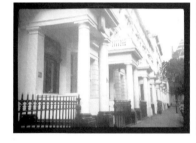

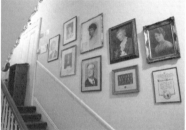

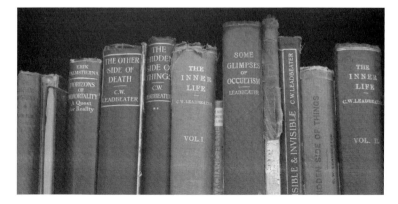

Foreword: Max Eames

With tears streaming down her cheeks, a middle-aged woman choked, "I *knew* it. Didn't I *say* so? See? Isn't it wonderful! A natural gift! That was *some* fireworks show. Just the beginning – and it *can't* stop here." Others were similarly moved, although one ashen-faced man had left our little windowless room because he felt "unsettled by it all."

But what had actually just happened?

All I knew was that I felt suddenly hungry. Ravenous. Starving, surely. "Drink some water, and then come with me." I had only just met Bunty; fiery and mercurial. And more than a bit 'Miss Jean Brodie', except well after her prime – 80-odd, I should think. Just the sort of person I'd instinctively saddle up to on a residential retreat jolly, before the inevitable storm-clouds of Day Two boredom filled the skies above me.

Bunty took me all the way down to the basement kitchens for a sandwich. "So I guess you're quite impressed with yourself? An *American* trait, is it? Just for the record, it's not you doing it, and it's nothing unique. Got it? I can see right through you like a sheet of glass… Here, drink more water – you're as high as a kite."

"I don't understand – what were they *talking* about, and why were they so moved?" Half an hour before, one of the facilitators had rescued me from falling asleep in a tedious lecture about something vaguely scientific. I'd been staring out the window for ages at the Hertfordshire countryside – this was an old convent, and to generate a bit of cash for the maintenance of their Neo-Gothic pile, the powers-that-be had allowed this "likeminded" retreat to take place.

I'd been ushered into an upstairs room, where a young woman was lying on a table with a blanket draped over her. It all struck me as a bit pre-rehearsed. There were four or five others besides Bunty in the room, all workshop presenters. Some I'd met; some I hadn't. One was a self-help author whose books I'd read voraciously. On locking eyes with him, I couldn't stop myself from blushing – I *hate* when that happens! He just grinned.

I was asked to put my hands over the woman's stomach and move up and down her body until I felt something like magnets – and then to see if I could find a few more. Which I'd dutifully set out to do, though only out of politesse. It felt weird.The 'magnets' were all in a line. I was encouraged to "trust my intuition" – or better yet, simply "trust." Eyes half-closed, my hands just went

7

where they wanted to go. They moved off that invisible line of 'magnets' to hover above various other parts of this woman's body. It wasn't at all embarrassing, though my hands were in places that would normally result in an uncontrollable blush-fest. And after a while it somehow felt as if it was over and done with, so I stopped. Clumsily. Then I opened my eyes – and turned crimson!

This was my first introduction to healing. I was just beginning to learn to "outgrow my illness" and refer to my various health issues since a child as "a friend who had come to teach me great truths." Yes, all the biopsies, the operations, the reconstructions, the humiliating years as a teenager, half of which were spent in a perpetual cycle of recovery – and in a wheelchair!

It's an absolute certainty that Bunty could read minds: "So, superstar, aside from feeling quite pleased with yourself, you're feeling sorry for yourself, too? We're going to have to do some work on that 'solar plexus' stuff – it's like a whirling dervish down there!"

Thus began my journey into the 'unseen world'. In hindsight, when the Board of Trustees of the College of Psychic Studies decided to refresh its Mission Statement, the strong focus on healing was at the forefront of my mind. It was somehow a deeply personal sense that the College is a 'beacon of light' – not just for those of us who've discovered it, but for many yet to come. What Bunty may have seen – but chosen not to tell me – was that illness was to "teach me great truths" for a very long time. After all, our true friends don't abandon us, do they? In my Lost Decade, where the only two things I could muster up the life-force to endure were the doctor and the College's healing clinics, I was what you'd call a 'regular'. Like a true friend, the clinics have always been there, rock-solid; I expect they always will.

It is a great pleasure to understand more about the depth and breadth of experience, dedication and personal growth that lay within the healing clinic groups. Many of us, in a time of need, forget to remind ourselves that to share the gift of healing represents an almost inconceivable act of generosity, the reward of connectedness between mind, body and spirit for which the College stands.

Max Eames
President, College of Psychic Studies

Introduction: Adam Price

This book is a testament to that spirit of fellowship engendered when people come together, perhaps share their troubles for a moment, and then put these behind them for a while. All of us can discover that excitement which comes through actually making a painting or writing a poem, also the enjoyment from seeing or hearing other people's creations.

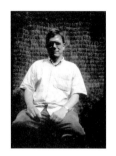

the**moment**is**now**! group sums up for me everything I love about Sunlight: the garden, the cafe, easy access for disabled members, the welcome in general. The Sunlight Centre has been an integral part of this project, as has the leadership and enthusiasm of Tina Lawlor Mottram.

Pinhole photograph of Adam Price relaxing in the garden at Sunlight
Photo by David Wise

Meditation has proved really powerful with this group. Members have found out more about about how mind and body are connected, and how healing can help. I understand that Gill and Rose have sometimes joined Tina and Win, as healers during sessions.

The group has looked at illness in a creative way - drawing and painting, auras, creative writing - and this has sometimes brought revelations to people. This book tells a number of stories from along the way. Everybody seems to have loved something from taking part in this project, whether it's the group meetings, the chat, the serious conversation.

Underlying all the little jokes: illness with a giggle! For once people have done the doing, not the doctors and the nurses. Enjoy the book....

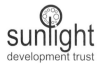

Adam Price
Trustee of Sunlight Development Trust
and
Treasurer of the**moment**is**now**!

Chapter 1:
Working creatively with long term illness, well being and health

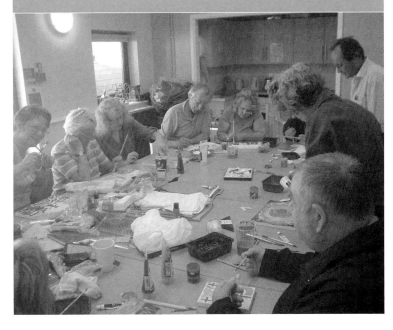

The creative group at work at Sunlight in July 2009

"I seek to inspire doctors and nurses to see that treating the person is as important, if not more so, than treating the disease itself."
Jonathon Hope

In world religions, mythology and folklore, the tree is a universal symbol for the inner directions of the cosmic process and its goal; the centredness of man and his world.
*Roger Cook, The Tree of Life [*1]*

themomentisnow

We are a group of artists, writers and healers working on projects about long term health: expressing the seen and unseen in words and image. Funded by Awards for All in 2009-10, this book records a year in the life of the project.

This story started a long time ago. It's difficult to pinpoint exactly when and where; visualise a seed of an idea that landed on some very fertile ground and started extending roots, with trust, into a welcoming Earth. For me, the story commences with trees. See it as the Tree of Life, rooted deep in the earth, with arms spread into the heavens and the sky, its broad trunk supporting its branches, leaves, flowers, fruit and all that lives on and near it. This idea of mine, supported by the healers at the College of Psychic Studies, Sunlight Development Trust and funded by Awards for All, has grown from seed to harvest and fruit, metaphorically this book. The idea germinated deep in winter with snow covering the frosty ground. The branches extended in summer, with autumn chasing colours and me to produce the fruit in time for spring the following year, so that the annual cycle may continue.

This is a story interwoven with many stories; not only of illness but also of well being and healing, of quiet spaces and time, of understanding and acceptance. The stories all somehow connect to the Wednesday Group Healing Clinic in the College of Psychic Studies, often only through me – a connector, a link between those with the illnesses, the carers, the creative instinct and then also me as a healer in the clinic. These stories are as rich as the tapestry of human lives and by sharing them, my role is defined as story teller of real lives and the very many people I have met during this project. All I can hope is that the way these people lives touched me will also touch you as you read.

The Tree of Life is a very ancient symbol. For the Maya, their precious Ceiba tree stood rooted at the very centre of everything, encompassing all worlds, seen and invisible. The roots represented the Underworld (of death, night, darkness), the trunk represented this world of the mundane and the branches soaring for the sky, reached into the Afterlife, the heavens and a skyworld of stars and deities. Buddha sheltered under a tree, escaping the midday sun. Adam was offered the fruit of the tree by the serpent, the apple of knowledge. He stole it and mankind's suffering is forever enshrined in this act of stealing the forbidden fruit. The tree and its fruit still offer us shelter, wisdom and joy for all seasons and weathers.

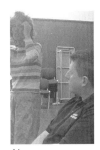

A group of people met early in the summer of 2009 in Gillingham in Kent, to set up a small support group that aimed to work creatively with long term illness. It included people who had long term medical conditions, along with their carers and sometimes family members and friends. Some people came along just to tell their story and to hear some of the others in the group. The group included some artists, some writers, a few healers, and some had come along just to see what would happen with the group. Many members had previously joined a support group and they were keen to see what would be different about this one.

Above: Lizz and Karl at the first meeting. Below: Charlie

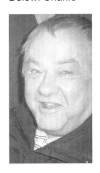

The tree idea blossomed and grew within the whole group. For some, it was a symbol of recovery from their illness. For others, it was a link to the natural world. In meditations, gradually the tree became a constant. In the group healing clinic, Greta, one of the healers visualised a tree with its branches full of light, standing in the centre of our clinic, in the space where we send our distant healing. The Tree of Light became the name of the project. Many of us found ourselves painting trees and flowers. Most of enjoyed the summer sunshine and the trees in the garden at Sunlight, where the project workshops took place. As summer turned to autumn, colours also changed hue. We continued our project as the leaves were falling, while friendships grew and various storylines began to emerge. The wonderful thing was that there was so little whingeing about being ill. There is only a limited amount of energy available to people with long term conditions and they know it. Energy can be used wisely, like a squirrel hiding nuts in autumn, for use in winter cold. So the group met and continued their painting and writing.

The roots are strong it seems. As this book celebrates almost a year of our lives, the participants are glad to have forged such a strong group and we very aware of the positive benefits it continues to bring to all our lives.

Conditions this group are dealing with:

Alcoholism
Aspergers Syndrome
ADHD
Bipolar Disorder
Cancer
Cerebellar Ataxia
Chronic Pain Syndrome
Damage to receptors in the brain
Depression
Diabetes Mellitus
Dyspraxia
Fibromyalgia
Kidney failure
Leukaemia
Osteoarthritis
Osteoporosis
Osteopenia
Psoriasis
Pernicious Anaemia
Post Traumatic Stress Disorder
Rheumatoid Arthritis
Temporo Mandibular Joint Disorder
Trigeminal Neuralgia
Carers and families of people with these conditions

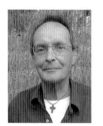

Above: Ken
Below: Adam

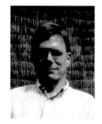

For more help and information about these conditions, please see Appendix 2, which includes support groups for some of the conditions.

Although not all these long term conditions were the same, we as a group have all learned a great deal by recognising some common areas of concern, and also by sharing when we meet up every few weeks. We have had moments of breakthroughs, of sadness, of tearful sharing and instants of great hilarity! There have been singing moments when we all burst into song in the garden at Sunlight in the sunshine. At times, Charlie has read us his poems aloud. While painting and writing, many people surprised themselves that actually they 'can paint!'

Meditation, healing and spirituality were an intrinsic

part of this project, and people who experience illness often want to explore the complementary 'holistic' route, in addition to the allopathic medical experience. The group has tried meditation at every meeting, often led by a different member of the group. It is agreed to be powerful by those who had never tried it before and the group experience seems to bring with it, an energy of its own.

As someone who has led quite a few of these meditations, I find a theme occurs to me as people walk into the room. There are up days and down days, some days with lots of people, others days with very few and usually I just concentrate on breathing in order to relax, followed by the chosen image. At times, others join in and add their piece and the idea grows. There have been some revelatory moments afterwards. On one occasion, two people experienced exactly the same image while meditating, with a very special meaning for both of them. This was shared, not on the day but at a later date, after they had discussed it among themselves. Meditation allows people time and space to delve deep into their own memory banks and beyond; our sessions have produced some "co-incidences", some insights and certainly everybody's creativity has been stimulated to produce their visual work afterwards. We have also made trips to the healing clinic in the college of Psychic Studies and healing has been offered at most meetings, time and space permitting. In fact, some of the people who are dealing with serious conditions themselves (Rose, Gill and Tina) have joined in with some healing and some Reiki when it was offered to Gordian, Ken and anybody who wanted some. This was a very special moment for us; sending healing energy and being joined by others in the group.

As a group, we have many limitations to their lives; the need to take medication long term brings with it side effects and complications. Sometimes you need to take drugs and then also other drugs to counteract the bad effect of the first ones on the body. People become very discerning in their choice of which drugs to take, balancing the pain relief aspect with the threat of addiction. One

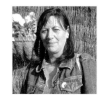

Above: Cathy
Below: Karen
*Photo by
Cerys Evans*

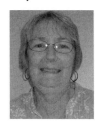

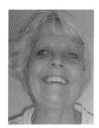

Above: Pat
Below: Gordian

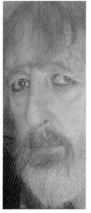

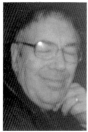

Above: Doug

member of the group weaned himself off morphine during the summer of 2009, with great difficulty and courage, because not to do so would have caused further damage to the receptors in his brain.

As members of our group have discovered, sometimes there is no medication, often there is not even a name for the illness; it is simply a matter of putting up with it. Diagnosis of the illness and of subsequent complications was high on the list of topics to discuss among the group as well as dealing with doctors, specialists and hospitals. The issue of being in pain (constantly, sometimes, often) and the ways people have adapted their lives around this was 'an eye-opener' according to Pat, one member of the group.

She journeyed with another group member to the healing clinic in London and was able to view first hand some of the limitations of being in a wheelchair. "I have met up with other people who have got health and social problems that are not fully being met by statutory providers. Meeting with these folk and getting them to tell their stories has been an eye opener of just what is out there (or not). I know that I have found the aspects of being with them, and going to the various creative art workshops, (art is not my best thing as I cannot draw for toffee) but specifically to London with one of our number, escorting him in his wheelchair on trains and taxis for our healing day, was something I would not have missed."

Another member of the group, Doug, describes his pain as "my jaw complaint is my alarm clock", explaining that it wakes him almost every day at a certain time. "The pain becomes unbearable when it travels up the facial nerve to the eye. I then get very confused as to the medication that best suits my degree of pain, as it could be a sinus problem, or a bout of Trigeminal Neuralgia." Doug's writing is in Chapter 5.

Although nature is often cited as a great healer, the natural world is not always beneficial for members of this group. The wind has featured many times in our discussions, as many members find it is a trigger for some of their conditions. Cold winds are listed as one of the factors which trigger attack for those that have jaw conditions eg Trigeminal Neuralgia and other conditions. Wind also affects mobility; strong wind becomes a real problem for some members of the group and many people with long term conditions feel unable to tackle public transport, with the frequent bus changes, the cold wind while waiting for the bus, the train transfers and so on and consequently, they often simply stay at home. This was very much the case in January 2010 in the snowstorms that brought the whole country to a standstill. There was great frustration for members of our group, some of whom were confined to their homes. 'I cannot go out. It's too dangerous. I am completely dependent on other people to help me' was one comment from our wheelchair user, Gordian.

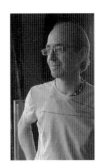

Above: Jonathon

However, one of the great things about this group is how members have tended to meet up and collect each other to get to the meetings, thereby banding together for support and also ensuring that people came regularly, as somebody else is depending on you so you go. In an early workshop, I asked people to visualise their pain as an animal and then on coming out of the meditation, I asked them to draw it or paint it. Gordian's image really is both primitive and scary. He has long, talon like nails. He is red and fiery and angry looking, with wild wings extending from his back. "This is my pain that lives in my body. Every day he drags it along my body. I take enough

Below: Gordian's Pain Animal, which can also be seen in the Colour Section.

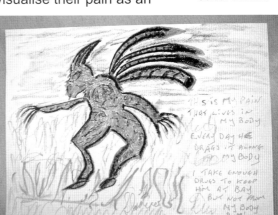

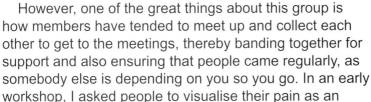

drugs to keep him at bay but not from my body. Bum!"

Then in a gesture to balance out the anger and pain and what I later learned is typical of Gordian, he drew "The Other Side." This picture is full of vivid orange flowers and a childlike sun. Somehow through his constant pain, he always manages to cheer other people up and make us laugh. He informs us that his lifestyle is why he is in pain and he knows it. See Gordian's story 'From 0 to 60' later in this chapter. A recent text comment from him was "Soon be Christmas, am disabled, slightly mad! But I'm alive to tell you!"

Doug, who has really difficult moments with jaw pain, comments "I have always maintained that my condition is as much about *relief* as the very pain itself. My pain could be identified as intermittent but I openly admire, those unlike myself, who are victims of constant pain." One of the few pieces of advice Doug could possibly offer to anyone with a long term condition is to immerse oneself into activities to take the mind off one's condition and to maintain a positive approach throughout.

For many of us, explaining our conditions and our needs was a topic for discussion. Communication brought up some very interesting issues for the group. Very few people with a long term condition seemed interested in moaning about what they couldn't do. It seems that a bitterly earned knowledge comes with a long term illness or condition: You only have a limited amount of energy. Most of the group were actively putting their energy into what they *could* do and also limiting their time to activities they enjoyed, whenever possible. At the start of the workshops, certain members of the group seemed to talk an awful lot, while others painted and experimented with writing.

I referred to what Dr Caroline Myss[*2] calls 'woundology' ie a public sharing of wounds as part of a support programme. However, Dr Myss doesn't believe that we are supposed to stay wounded. She argues that we are meant to move through our tragedies and challenges and to help each other through the many painful episodes in our lives. In her book 'Why people don't heal and how they can' Dr Myss posits that wounds are the means through which we enter the hearts of other people; teaching us to be compassionate and wise. Gill and her husband Derrick, and their family, have experienced a lot of ill health. However, at one of our group meetings it became clear that the family had never had the time, space and opportunity to fully appreciate some of how coping with illness had transformed them in ways unimaginable. I had asked the group to look at a few questions.

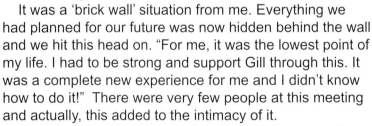

- What is your story?
- What good has come of it?
- What were your lowest moments?
- What advice can you offer for people with long term conditions?

When you are a close family unit, I guess the sharing of that with an external person was quite illuminating. Derrick was busy writing his piece and commented that he had never stopped to think about it before. Here is his story.

Derrick Solly's story
The 'Brick Wall'

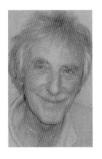

My wife Gill has suffered from a rare neurological condition called Cerebellar Ataxia all her life. (See Gill's story later in this chapter.) We have been married for 37 years. About 11 years ago, her condition worsened and we took the decision to take early retirement from my career as an engineer to become my wife's carer. 5 years ago, she was diagnosed with cancer.

It was a 'brick wall' situation from me. Everything we had planned for our future was now hidden behind the wall and we hit this head on. "For me, it was the lowest point of my life. I had to be strong and support Gill through this. It was a complete new experience for me and I didn't know how to do it!" There were very few people at this meeting and actually, this added to the intimacy of it.

Derrick realised that even while ill, Gill was supporting him because she knew that he was floundering. She knew that he needed his strength to continue to care for her. His open admiration for Gill was simply humbling to behold. "Help came from an unexpected source. It was Gill herself!" James, their son, who was also at the meeting was nodding in agreement. It really was a very tender moment for everybody and for the family, it was a release and an ability to analyse the past without getting very morbid about it, just acknowledgement that they had been through it and come out stronger as a result.

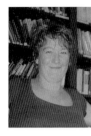

Sarah Jenkin's story
The 'Magic Word'

Hi, my story is all about how one jaw being put out of joint can really throw you! Last year I couldn't walk the length of myself. The world spun around me and my feet felt like they would give from under me. This they call 'vertigo'. Such a small word for such a big shock. Except it shouldn't have been such a shock, and it wasn't, once I started looking back. For the two years beforehand, my whole body was beginning to close in on itself, starting from my head downwards like someone pulling the strings on a doll too tight. I'd been having problems with my jaw and pain and tinnitus, but no-one seemed to think they could do anything about it. The magic word "stress" was mentioned a few times and that, it seemed, was it.

Once the magic word is mentioned nothing else can be done. But the pain in the jaw was the worst. I knew that if there was a problem, it was there. The dentist didn't know what to do. The GP uttered the magic word (Stress) so that left me to the quacks. Acupuncture, Bowen, reflexology, even an osteopath. Nothing seemed to shift it. Do whatever you can about stress when a pain becomes bad and nothing seems to shift it, it starts to get you down. But eventually the vertigo kicked in. So off to the GP who was helpful in terms of drugs, which were given for each successive diagnosis. Not this? Try this! You're young for vertigo, aren't you?

Could this be related to the pains in my jaw, neck, head? I asked. None of the other drugs you've given me seem to work, and it is worse when I touch that area. My dentist had diagnosed me with TMJ Disorder (Temporo Mandibular Joint Disorder) and after some online investigation and www.patient.co.uk, I found some info.

Of course this was a bad move, I'm not medically trained so what do I know? Eventually the pain was so bad I asked for muscle relaxants and the GP, to shut me up, gave them to me. These did the trick, of course, but once I started to cut back, the problem returned. There was only one person I knew dealt with this. So, back to the osteopath. Oh yes, he said, you get vertigo with jaw problems like yours. Didn't you know? It's very common.

What good (if any) has come out of it?

To be honest the time I have been ill is time wasted, and time wasted for no good reason. I am very angry that I wasn't listened to, I am angry I am still dealing with the side effects of the medicines I have been given and angry I had to pay for my own treatment. I am angry that the magic word "stress" was used as an excuse not to take my concerns seriously. As a result, my tolerance for timewasters and bullshitters has lowered considerably.

Being a nice girl and taking my medicine without complaining got me absolutely nowhere. It proved to me that although medical staff are hardworking and mean well, they are not infallible. It also proved to me that I have the capacity to keep going and the strength of will to find the information myself, and the people to get the right treatment. But more positively, I did go to one of your painting sessions. I haven't done any painting before, and certainly not done any artistic work with colour since school. It was fun to just play and not worry about how "good" the picture was or if it was right. It was liberating to do something because it was fun.

Your lowest moments?

Crying in frustration because I couldn't walk the length of myself without the world spinning round me. Being told it was all in my head and I should just get over my "stress" and everything would be okay. Not being believed or even listened to, especially when I mentioned this to my family who at first were sure I was "putting it on". Having to negotiate the paperwork at work, feeling ashamed at being off when they were having problems with staffing levels. Generally feeling ashamed at being so "weak" and stupid for not getting it fixed earlier. I was prescribed tranquillisers by one particular specialist, who didn't even bother to ask me what my symptoms were before he diagnosed me, the magic word again: S –T –R –E –S –S, and complained about me making him late for his lunch. All this trouble because of one dickey jaw. The arrogance of the man was staggering. I laugh about it now, of course, because I am being treated by someone competent.

I managed to find myself someone who would treat the jaw on a permanent basis, as good as the osteopath is, he is really only plugging the leaks. Patrick Grossmann in London (who bothered to examine me) asked me what my symptoms were, confirmed the thing about the vertigo and basically got on with treating me. My jaw does make weird clicking noises still but the pain is gone. And no more vertigo.

Any advice for other people with long term illness?
"Arm yourself with knowledge, but be careful about the sources you use. Use the library. Connect with people online, there will be a support group there if there isn't one locally, but be careful about the sites you use. Ask yourself who the person is who posted the information, where they got it from, why you believe them. Is it appropriate for you, and does it answer your question. Why do you believe them? In fact, ask that about any medical advice you get, no matter what the source.

The TMJ forum online helped me to understand what was going on with my body and helped me to locate the person who is treating me now. Without that knowledge I wouldn't have had the treatment, or the massive improvement I have had in my condition now. It isn't 100 per cent and possibly never will be, and I haven't finished my treatment yet. But I know there are people I can talk to now who will understand what I am going through and offer practical advice."

Communication issues were often seen as causing stress for the members of the group, often because of the lack of knowledge from the general public (and sometimes also medical professionals); this was a frequent topic of debate in between daubs on a canvas. Sometimes the conditions had no medical test or name or it was simply outside the scope of an ordinary GP, whose job is general medicine, not to be a specialist or expert in every illness. Support groups can be helpful for some members, if they exist at all. However, as Cerebellar Ataxia is a little known condition, Gill, one of our members, has had to set up her own support group for people with this very rare condition.

Ataxia is a very rare neurological disorder, which causes muscle wasting, and in turn affects mobility and movement. It also affects sight, hearing, speech, and can cause serious fatigue. There are two main types of Ataxia: Cerebellar Ataxia and Friedrich's Ataxia, both of which can affect both men and women of any age, including children. There is no known treatment. Two members of our creative group have Ataxia and their family have also attended. Gill Solly founded her own support group, in St Margaret's and St Peter's church in Rochester, as none existed.

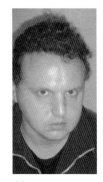

Above: James, Gill and Derrick's son, who helps at Gill's group

Below: Gill, who set up her own support group for Cerebellar Ataxia

Gill Solly's story

"Cerebellar Ataxia affects everything, it is progressive, your movement is bad – and it can only get worse!" says Gill. Even speaking is a problem, as the condition affects the clearness of speech and often "people assume you are stupid, people don't even try to understand you." See poems by Gill Solly and Ray Moxon on this theme later in this book. Gill has had a lot of mourning in her life, in addition to coping with her own rare illness. Her mother died in childbirth and Gill was born 20 minutes later. Gill describes how Ataxia paralysed her left side, from the neck down. 'I was a delicate child' and she had a lot of problems at school, due to her disability. 'No kid should go through what I went through' Gill says, as she describes being bullied, because she was unable to do various physical activities such as PE. Gill's Nan, Constance, who became the carer of Gill and her siblings with her husband Jim, was told not to hold out too much hope for Gill. However,

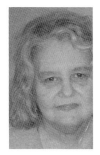

Gill survived and despite being told, later in life, that she wouldn't be able to have children she has proved medical opinion wrong. It seems that Gill has a great determination to live life and live it to the best of her ability. She now has 3 boys with her husband Derrick.

Gill became pregnant with a girl, who died shortly after birth. On top of dealing with a chronic long term health condition, Gill felt this was all too much. We spoke at length in our creative group about losing a child. It seems unnatural in the order of things. No parent expects to lose a child before they go themselves. During a discussion in the group, it emerged that many members of the group had lost a child or a partner. 4 women and 1 man in this small group had lost a child. The frank conversations while painting were refreshing to hear. People who had been through numbing loss were able to chat over a cup of tea and a splash of colour on a canvas about their feelings. All of the group who spoke on this theme submitted a poem for this book on the subject, which you can read in Chapter 5. Below Gill describes how she lives with Ataxia.

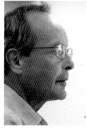

Above: Ken

Ataxia, Ataxia **Gill Solly**

Ataxia, ataxia,
What is this thing ataxia?
I don't understand it, it is so rare,
There is no cure, no medical care.
and my speech is impaired.

I feel all alone with it, and so tired am I
my muscles are weak,
I cannot walk straight.
The stairs look like Everest,
I climb them each night.

My hands shake so much,
a tossed salad I prepare.
The trouble, you see,
is the Cerebellum is wrong,

that part of the brain
the messages come from.
The messages travel through
the nerves and the muscles,
but they don't reach my feet.

Ataxia, ataxia, people stare,
they don't understand,
they're just not aware.
You must bring awareness,
we must help each other,
If you have this diagnosis,
or problems like this,
You're not alone;
we're here to care.

I've lived with this illness for 56 years,
So I understand what you're going through,
My family and I, 12 years ago
set up this group, for people like
me and you, to go.

We share a meal and a chat,
our friendship is strong,
so give me a ring (e-mail as well),
or just come along.
Bring your family and friends,
and all will be well.
So you can phone me any day,
I'm here to help in any way.

Roy Moxon's story
I first met Roy at Gill Solly's Ataxia Friendship Group – see Index 2 for details. When I met Roy and Ann, he was very concerned that I wouldn't understand his speech and he seemed quite surprised by how quickly the condition had made him lose his ability to speak and to write and all the things that people consider 'normal'. His diagnosis had been very recent; unlike Gill his had developed later in life.

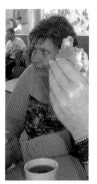

Below: Jane in Cafe Sunlight

Roy and his wife came to the art group only once and my lasting memory of him was his smile. I had visualised a meditation with clouds. I really wanted people who had mobility problems to enjoy being healthy. Feeling light and weightless and airy, and able to view the world from a high vantage point. When they opened their eyes, I asked people to paint what they saw. Roy beamed at me and reported 'You know I can't speak and I can't cook. I can't write anymore but I can paint!' He was quite gleeful and he painted the clouds with joy at what he *could* do. In our comments book, his wife had written "Thoroughly enjoyed our first art class. Good to meet new friends."

Sadly, Roy passed away in November 2009, shortly after this art session. This is his poem.

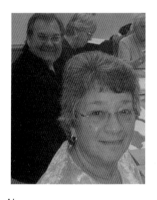

Above:
Roy and his wife Ann, who joined Gill's group in 2009. In the background, Win and Pat at work.

Roy's Ataxia **Roy Moxon**

My name is Roy, I'm 63.
I've led a busy life.
Got 2 kids and 4 grand kids.
And my carer is my wife.

Recently diagnosed with Ataxia
What is that? I hear you say.
Never heard of it.
I hear this every day.

Late onset cerebellar.
My type I'm told is pure.
There is no medication
Alas, there is no cure.

It affects my speech and balance
I find it difficult to walk
But when I've had a drink or two
You should hear the way I talk.

To my grandchildren I'm granddad

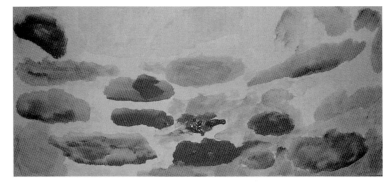

Left:
Clouds by
Roy Moxon.

The one with wobbly legs
I don't do any cooking
But they would love my scrambled eggs

I take one day at a time
No one knows what lies ahead
So when the morning comes around
It is worth getting out of bed.

I joined an Ataxia Friendship Group.
Our chat and thoughts we share.
It's nice to know you're not alone.
These people really care.

So if I'm feeling down one day.
Thinking Why? What if? Why me?
I'm grateful for my Ataxia friends
For all the laughs and cups of tea.

Mourning the loss of a loved one is a human heart
ache that most people experience in their lifetime,
illness or not. It is recognised that it takes time to heal and
that eventually, time does heal all. In this group, it seemed
there was a lot of silent mourning. 4 women and 1 man in
the group had lost children. Statistically this probably could
fit the normal average but it seemed a huge number when
looking round our table. This truly was a healing moment
for Lizz, who had lost her daughter Rosie, aged 6. Lizz

believed that it was this that had plunged her into deep depression and this was followed by the loss of her brother a few years later.

In a group meeting in the summer, I received an email from Lizz with the most touching piece of writing and I rejoiced that Lizz was coming through her dark patch and shedding some light upon it. Somehow the ball started rolling at one of our workshops. I suppose we always try to live in the present as much as possible. Mourning is a grieving process and it inevitably links people to the past and if this is a very painful past, then it may not be constructive after a long period. Sometimes people don't realise that they are actually able to move on.

Lizz Daniel's story

Lizz described how she listened in to a conversation at

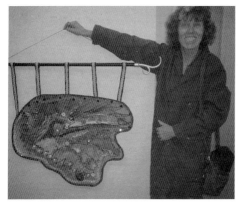

Lizz, holding her wall hanging, created from a recycled sheet and lots of imagination in 2009

one our July workshops. "Tina had brought along pastels watercolours and acrylics and was encouraging us all to be creative. I've been playing around with an unusual medium, (sticky back plastic) for years, so when Tina spread out the variety of paints, I was immediately stumped. What to do? Charlie resisted immediately and said he wanted to write a poem. "Fine" Tina replied, "Do what feels best for you." Poems, I pondered on the idea, and thought perhaps I could write a poem too, so after playing sponta-neously with some gorgeous black charcoal I wrote a little poem about depression. Charlie was telling us all about the poems he had written and wondered if they could be included in the book or put up on the website. "I've got a load of poems too," I piped up, "I wrote loads of stuff when Rosie my 6 year old daughter died."

Tina was silent for a moment. "What about writing something about how you are feeling *now*?" she said. "This book is all about what's going on in you now. Of course, the past bears some relevance but how are you coping today?" I thought about the poem I had just written about how my inner light was hidden away and realised it was based in the past and this rather threw me. What to do then? Looking around I saw that Gordian was slapping acrylic on to a piece of sheet Tina had brought along, and was teasing the paint in all directions. It looked fun.

Taking a large square of sheet, I began to play with the paint, wetting the material and spreading it on. It was messy but a delightful 'hands on' experience and I loved doing it. I wasn't that impressed with my end result but thought I might do a bit more at home. I had no idea what it was or what it might turn into, if anything at all. Once at home, I put it over the back of a chair where I could look at it. It stayed there for days. One morning after I had just got up and was on my way to the kitchen I passed it by and saw a shape emerging so immediately cut it out and left it there hoping for more inspiration. None came.

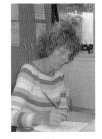

Above: Lizz
Below: Charles

Later that day my daughter popped in and commented that she liked what I had done. Funny when someone gives you a compliment about something, particularly her, as she's a hard one to please, it made me take a bit more notice and gave me a nice little boost. I looked at it with a different intent. Since the meeting I had been thinking a lot about where I was in my life and how I was coping with depression. I have been a depressive since a child of 8 when I lost my mother in a car accident overnight. She went out and never returned. In 1961 there was no bereavement counselling for kids and I grew up in a totally dysfunctional family environment that left its mark.

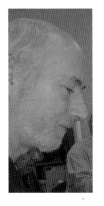

Low self-esteem and abandonment followed me through my life and I had many dark periods that I realise now was severe depression. The death of my 6 month baby son did nothing to help and increased terribly the feelings of guilt that I had grown up with. It wasn't until Rosie, the light of my life, died in 1996 of sudden meningitis, that I was able to begin a healing process that is still continuing today. Rosie's death took me to the darkest places I have been, the black abyss of despair a void that felt utterly hopeless where I was totally alone, yet it also allowed for healing to take place. I cried every day for a year, kept a journal and wrote loads of letters stories and poems.

Slowly I began to surface. I sought loads of help from many different agencies and began to heal ome of the wounds, but the depression was always there, lurking in the back of my mind, catching me unawares and spiralling me down into that dark familiar place I had grown up with. I still had a long way to go but knew I was rising and I began to seek healing from a variety of alternative sources.

Synchronicity became my friend and through various findings and investigations I became more aware of the interrelated connectedness of all things and my part in them. In the spiritual worlds it's called tragedy conscious-ness and without a doubt Rosie's death was a wake up call from God / divine being / universal intelligence / all that is. There was a point soon after my brother died on Christmas Eve 1999, when quite suddenly I birthed my creative spirit. I'm sure his death had something to do with it, and I'm sure he was guiding me. One day I just started making pictures with all the bits I had been collecting for years. Just like that, I started being creative and could not stop; it was the beginning of where I am now. Art has kept me sane, without a doubt, it lifted me up from the black hole, occupied and soothed my mind with pleasure; pushed away the pain, and led me forwards. That's how I came to meet Tina and that's how I came to be involved with this whole group. That's how I happened to make the bright painted blob that was lying on my living room floor.

So where was I now on this road of recovery? What was I going to do with this strange piece of artwork that had come out of nowhere? Ask and it shall be given - I'm working a lot with the law of attraction these days - and suddenly the universe provided me with the answer. Quickly I went down my workspace and started jazzing it up, sparkles and glitter, glue gun, sewing machine, needle and thread. This was something different; it felt good to be working in a different medium. Over the next few days it began to take shape but I still wasn't sure of what it was. I knew I liked it but there were still some gaps. Tina had planned a visit to the College of Psychic Studies for a group healing session that turned out to be a wonderful experience, really uplifting and rich in new vibrations. On my return home, I began to do more work on my piece. Suddenly I knew what I was playing with and got very excited for it fitted perfectly with where I was and how I felt. My work was a BURST OF JOY. I had grown into joy.

Next morning I woke up and was driven to rewrite the small poem I had initially begun that came about from the dark charcoal drawing, it's called

Somewhere Deep Inside
Lizz Daniels

Somewhere deep inside
Is a small spark
Of light
Yearning to be free.
Once I thought it was blocked,
Bound in pain and despair
But now I know
There are no blocks.
Nothing stands in the way
Between joy and me.
It is my birthright.
And the small spark
Once well hidden
Spins through the universe
Of My being,
Shining in the darkness
Contagiously igniting
Every cell
In my body
Paving the way
For love.

"Actually putting a name on it is very liberating and has

inspired me to do a series of similar work all depicting joy, which I am actively engaged in at present. I would never have thought that such a revelation would occur through an off the cuff piece of art made with no conscious intention whatsoever. Thanks Tina for helping me make the connection to joy." Since this moment, Lizz has assimilated the experience into a poem and moved on. She has gone back to study art at college, invigorated by her new found joy and trying to hold onto it when the clouds land on her shoulders.

For Win, who is a poet, carer and a healer, a crucial moment came for her on this project. Seeing her aura on screen, in August 2009 in Sunlight brought a new development to her own understanding of herself. This project had set out to explore illness in many ways and part of the project was the opportunity to see your aura. An aura is the energy field that surrounds the body, not visible to most human eyes. There are psychics and healers who can see them and healers work with this energy, often unable to see it but certainly sensitive to it. However, the ability to see auras is very rare. For a more detailed discussion about auras and their interpretation, please see Chapter 4. Win decided to try to write about how she lost her son to illness. Here is her story.

Win Gibbon's story
Everyone is entitled to the same respect
While on this project, Win decided to write about her son's condition, offering her experience and advice as a mother who has lost a son needlessly.

My son David died of Hodgkin's disease in 1997, which is a cancer affecting the immune system. He was diagnosed some 23 months before his death and would have made a full recovery from the disease, which is both treatable and curable, had he not been ignored by his GP surgery who branded him as being 'attention seeking' and who told him to 'go off and start living his life.'

The surgery had no knowledge of the disease or its symptoms and instead of referring him to the hospital, left

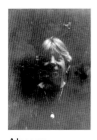

Above:
Pinhole photo
of Win by
David Wise

him to suffer through the first three stages of the illness. He attended a chest clinic for recurring bronchitis, where they recognised the symptoms immediately. There he was diagnosed, but he was at stage four, and not much could be done for him. He underwent surgery to remove certain glands, which were infected and then endured an aggressive course of chemotherapy. His last treatment before his death was a stem cell transplant, which was ineffective.

What have I learned from it?

When you are ill, the GP is the first person you go to, primarily to seek medication or advice on how to treat your condition, then ultimately to be referred to the hospital, if all else fails. In my son's case, this never happened and the anger I felt at the lackadaisical attitude of the GP's surgery still stays with me. My son was a colourful character who defied convention and lived and dressed as he pleased with body piercing and hair the colour of the rainbow, when it wasn't destroyed by the ravages of chemotherapy and I think his appearance played an important part on his treatment at the GP surgery. They treated him in a different light and nobody should ever be judged by their appearance and attitude to life. Everyone is entitled to the same respect.

Jonathon, a member of our creative group, has a camera, hand sensors and equipment, which can record auras. He had offered to do aura photos with members of the group, also giving them some interpretation. Jonathon has worked in this area as a result of his own illness and it can seem like a magic show, as an image of a person shows on the screen and subsequently, colours appear. Like everybody else, Win stared at the screen and saw almost complete white, which apparently, is really very unusual.

"Jonathon told me my aura was pure white, which indicated that I had angels present. I could identify with this because I've had reason to believe that my son could be my spirit guide." Win is a Reiki healer and she writes that "this experience confirmed a lot of the feelings I've had about myself." Shortly afterwards, Win wrote a poem looking at the time of year when her son passed away, which is still a trigger for memories. See Win's poem in Chapter 5.

"When Jonathon told me that my aura was pure white, which indicates that I had angels present in my healing plane, I could identify with this. I've had reason to believe that my son could be my spirit guide. He has been seen at a healing session I've attended."

Lowest moments

My lowest moments always come just before Christmas. My son died on the 10th of December and that day still lives with me as if it were yesterday. He was married and lived with his wife and family about 70 miles from me, so I didn't experience all the pain and suffering of my lovely son. I was saved from all that. But I still recall that fateful day when that telephone call urged me to make that 70 mile dash along the motorway to sit with him because they didn't think he would last the night but as I walked into the room, he died.

Advice for others with longterm conditions
• Cry when you want to
• Get as many hugs as you can fit in
• Walk your heart out
• Swim your lungs out
• Laugh your head off
• And if you've got any part of your body left after this, look after it!

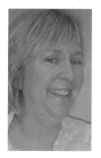

Above: Lily, Cerys and Roxy
Below: Beverley

Beverley Evans' story

During the holidays I went along to Sunlight, where I was able to participate in an art session using proper paints and a canvas. When I got there I was with 3 children, aged 6 and under, and I felt very tense and hyper vigilant. My concern was to offer my daughter Cerys and her friends a lovely opportunity to paint and chat and play and socialise, which they did. Incredibly, within minutes of Tina placing a canvas in front of *me* and sitting me down, I began to paint and something wonderful happened.

I loved it. I sat completely involved in my canvas and I

couldn't believe how quick and easy it was to lose myself and allow myself to focus on me and my thoughts.
What (if anything) have you learned from it?
It's not easy to say but really I loved being in my head and painting it let me do that. Sitting, looking at the canvas, and thinking about the colours, the paint thickness and thinness, the lines and shapes and patterns.
Lowest moments?
I always avoid being in my own thoughts. I am always too busy or too tired or too distracted. Like many people, I avoid this. Why I am not sure but truthfully I guess it's lonely.
The healing experience
My own experience with healing is quite a strong physical reaction. Initially as I sit upright and calm, I feel nauseous and dizzy almost like my body resisting to it and I have to fight to make myself absorb the calm and peace. I find the experience intense and completely worthwhile.

I have had the chance to experience healing sessions for myself but my real comments have to be about the healing sessions I witnessed at my school. I had arranged for a healer to come into the school. The young people who attend my school, experience social emotional and behavioural difficulties, and are usually tense loud and unable to relax, listen to others or communicate.

I, and my colleagues, were amazed as we witnessed our students engage and respond to the healing in ways we might never have imagined. Facial expressions completely changed. One young man on the autistic spectrum (ASD) came out and was not only calm and relaxed but smiling, something he rarely does and the next day he reported to going home and sleeping! His mother could not believe it. Other students reported feeling electricity and were able to verbalise feelings and emotions around anger in a very descriptive and informative way.

Sometimes, illness sets you on a new wave of learning experience, often challenging your strongly held beliefs. It amazes me how positive most of the people on this project are; no matter how tough the journey has been.

Jonathon Hope's story

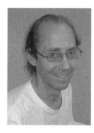

In my late teens I was diagnosed with kidney failure. This meant that without lifelong treatment, I would die. Since then, over the last 30 years, it has felt like I have experienced pretty much everything that ill health could throw at me. In fact, sometimes it felt like I was clinging onto life by my fingernails alone and until relatively recently, I suffered unimaginably.

Kidney failure itself meant enduring symptoms that made life a daily struggle, 18 years of dialysis, innumerable operations, years of hospitalisation and 4 transplants. It was will power alone that got me through most of it. Most of the time I was dragging my body kicking and screaming behind me. However, in the latter part of this journey, with the help of many, including family, friends, healthcare professionals and an extraordinary team of healers and mediums, I have healed myself. I now feel fully recovered.

In contrast to the medical consensus, I truly believe this transplant will never fail. After a tremendous amount of inner work, I have reconnected with a lightness of being, a joy, a sense of fun and peace that I could never previously have dreamed of. Physically, emotionally and spiritually, I have never felt better.

What good has come out of it?

So much good has come out of it that it is hard to cover it all. Firstly, as a person I am very different to when I first started on this journey of ill health. I used to always be strictly rational, logical, self-centred, fearful and in my brain. However, now I am more guided by my intuition, my inner wisdom and my heart. I now feel more compassionate, empathetic and loving of others and even of myself. I am a lot less fearful and life itself is now a blessing.

Secondly, I am now much more open-minded and without that, I believe I would not have fully recovered. I now accept that I have the power to overcome my illness and all its symptoms. I now accept that healing can make a real difference to one's health. I now accept that there is profound meaning in disease.

Thirdly, I now no longer see my illness as just another example of unimaginable, overwhelming and needless suffering. Rather I see it as a gift. A gift of experience with which I can now help others who face similar challenges. As a result, I regularly speak out at medical conferences, write articles in medical journals and seek to inspire doctors and nurses to see that treating the person is as important, if not more so, than treating the disease itself.

Lowest Moments?

Being diagnosed with such an irrevocable, life-long illness such as kidney disease is a body blow to the system. It is like walking into a brick wall. It disempowered me utterly, decisions were made on my behalf by others with little reference to my own wishes. For a long initial period, my natural coping strategy was to simply close myself down from life itself. From friends, family, loved ones as well as society. I simply endured. My hopes and dreams went out of the window. The amount of pain, needless pain was unimaginable. I was not happy, comfortable, at ease or enjoying life. But I was alive.

The single toughest moment in my life was observing, on an overhead monitor, my third transplant fail during a CT scan and the subsequent coma, paralysis, and inability to talk or move. It took me nine months to get back on my feet and get out of hospital. Strangely, despite all this, I never lost hope. Intriguingly, this, my most harrowing experience, was to prove my lifeline and a so-called Near Death Experience, together with a firm decision that I wanted to change myself, proved to kick start a powerful inner awakening. In time, this helped utterly transform my life and well-being for the better.

This group has shared many collective experiences connected to being ill on a longterm basis. At our very first meeting Nigel declared "We are the experts in our conditions. In this room, we have more expertise than the whole medical profession in Medway!" It is knowledge from being a 'patient', and dealing with all that goes with that. Stress varied from simple things like getting the right prescription *regularly* to transport, carers and getting the right support. Regular medication frequently involves going to the GP to order it, then taking it 2 days later to the chemist and frequently having to go back to collect the prescription the following day. Sometimes when you do go back to collect it, there is a mistake. And this is every month of every year for the rest of your life. Sure, it keeps you alive but it would be good to have a medication holiday once in a while. Being ill often seems to be a full time job, as many people in this group would agree.

From making hospital appointments, to getting drugs, to dealing with social services, benefits due and needed. Being ill on a long term basis is difficult enough; however, it often seems to include being quite poor, as many people either quit work due to illness or to look after their partner. This results in having to battle with social services for help, both physical and financial. One member of the group who uses a wheelchair, found that his mobility allowance was 'checked' for him by an official.

Subsequently, it was discovered that he had been 'overpaid' and his allowance was cut back so that his carer could not come for 3 days anymore. "When you are ill, you don't feel up to dealing with all this paperwork" he said with resignation.

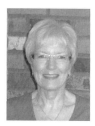

Photo by
Tony Mardel

Jean Mardel's story
Living with Trigeminal Neuralgia
Until 1999, like most people I had never heard of Trigeminal Neuralgia. I had recently had quite a bit of dental work carried out which included some root canal treatment. When I had an attack of excruciating pain on the right side of my face I thought it was related to my teeth and was fortunate enough to get an appointment with my dentist within the hour. The poor man was faced with a patient begging him to find the cause of the pain

but not allowing him to touch their face. Somehow he came to the conclusion that there was nothing amiss with my teeth and recommended that I see an ENT Consultant and in the meantime, take the strongest pain killers available. These didn't touch the pain at all and my best means of treatment was to not move my face at all. This meant no talking, no eating; in fact, no movement or touching of my face. The attacks, when they occurred, were like having a live electric cable put on my skin; torturous. They may have only lasted a minute or two but it felt like a life time.

I had a private appointment with an ENT Consultant as there was no way I could wait to go down the NHS route. He identified my problem as Trigeminal Neuralgia, which is caused by pressure on the trigeminal nerve. This nerve has three branches; one which runs above the eye, the forehead and front of the head, the second runs through the cheek, upper jaw, teeth and gum and side of the nose and third which runs through the lower jaw, teeth and gum. Having prescribed a drug called 'Tegretol' to relieve the pain; he referred me to a Neurologist. The Consultant I saw was involved with the Trigeminal Neuralgia (TN) Association and understood the pain I was experiencing.

At first 'Tegretol' controlled the pain although it made me tired, affected my memory, slowed down my reactions and thought patterns and I feel changed my personality. I started on what was to be a pattern of life for the next five years, taking enough medication to control the pain, reducing this slowly when I had periods of remission, reoccurrences of neuralgia, back on the tablets, each time needing to reach a higher dose before the pain was controlled. I learned to avoid situations that may bring on an attack; going out on a windy day (the wind across my face would be a trigger), eating food that needed chewing, late nights and stress. I had been informed about the various treatments available apart from medication.

These were; gamma knife which uses radiation on the nerve and does not require anaesthetic, percutaneous rhizotomy, carried out under local anaesthetic - the surgeon makes tiny cuts in the side of the face and cuts or 'blocks' the trigeminal nerve by laser surgery, freezing or cauterisation and cranial surgery – microvascular decompression (MVD). I really thought I could beat this illness without having any of these and carried on with medication. As time went by, things were getting unbearable. Some days the pain would be around my mouth and I couldn't eat, drink or talk. My weight decreased and I felt desperately tired and ill. Other times the pain was across my head and around my eye, always on the right side of my face. I had to face the truth that I had to have surgery, this was no way to live and it was affecting my family and everyone around me.

My Consultant referred me to a specialist at Kings who arranged another MRI scan. This confirmed the fact that a blood vessel was resting on the nerve just behind my right ear. He went through the various options open to me and explained what the operation entailed, which was having a circle of bone removed from my head just behind my right ear so that the surgeon could separate the blood vessel and nerve then replace the bone.

I decided to have the operation as I felt that this was most likely to be successful. The weeks I waited for a hospital bed seemed interminable. By this time the pain was intense and I was at my wits end. My medication was changed from Tegretol to Gabapentin which did offer relief for a short while. At last I received the letter with my date of admittance. I was extremely nervous at the thought of the operation but also desperate to get rid of the pain and lead normal life.

Following the operation I spent a day in Intensive Care before being transferred on to the main ward where I stayed for about five days before being allowed home. Unfortunately I developed an infection and was readmitted for ten days. My recovery was slow and it was three months before I felt ready to return to work. Although MVD is not a pleasant procedure I did get immediate relief from neuralgia and enjoyed 5 pain free years. Unfortunately it has returned and I am now on medication again. As before, I try to avoid any situations that may aggravate the neuralgia and realise that the day may come when I have the MVD operation again. I certainly won't wait until I am at such a low point before do so this time.

During my illness I have found the Trigeminal Neuralgia Association to be a great support and receive regular new letters which give information on new developments and drugs plus articles from fellow sufferers. The TNA Association has a web site which gives information on the illness and treatments and details of how to join the association. It has now enlarged its remit to include all facial pain as there are many other conditions which have this effect. (See Index 2 for contact details.) I recommend any fellow sufferer to make contact.

Gordian Bailey's story:
From 0 to 60 in 6 decades
• **1950**
Born 5th of January. First 18 months cared for by "Auntie" Violet and "Uncle" Arthur, not living with parents, Ward of Court. Then with parents until aged 4, parents separated. Lived with paternal grandparents, Nellie and George, during term time. School holidays lived with maternal grandmother and "Uncle" (Lodger? Hmmm). Drinking buddy (of) Uncle Tom. 9 years and parents after long divorce battle – re marry? Only way Mum could gain formerly denied access! Lived with tempestuous mother and nasty father, called me 'idiot bastard son'. Great.

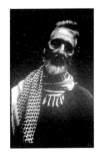

Pinhole photograph of Gordian by David Wise 2009

• **1960**
Aged 10, pretty good, no parental guidance or "caring life". Parents worked. I kept out of the way. Did jive with Mum. Not allowed to call her Mum! Reason, her age. Oops, not good. Father always, always at work.
Aged 11; off to Australia so my mother and her father can argue in a hot country! Learned shooting, surviving, surfing, living rough in scrubland – came back before my 16th birthday – October '65. Still a Ward of Court! October '65.
Finish with education (ha!). Bought fast motorcycle 250

41

Royal Enfield. Rubbish but "mine". Started to work at Acorn Shipyard, base of a new Medway Steam Packet Co. Discovered girls.

17 Girlfriend Carol was pregnant.

18 Left shipyard. Work for Medway Conservency Board (Later MPA).

27th of April 1968 Married Carol Cotter. 14th of October 1968 Nicola Annette Bailey born! Had our bedsit, then mad flat over shop. Discovered drugs!!

• 1970

Loads of freedom, fun time, still worked. Always off to gigs with Nicola (Nikki) and without. My parents now cope with having a grand-daughter? Still working, marine salvage.

1975

Father divorced mother, went back to Australia with new wife Coreen, with 2 lovely teenage sons, took all money in dvorce on grounds that my mother "unstable" mental health record and her being gay!

Kai born. Wow a son, brilliant. By end of decade, redundant. Carol and I divorced, Carol had met someone else. Carol 36, lover 18. Shame, gave me council house and 2 lovely children. Aged 28, single parent, two children, gave up work.

• 1980

Change of lifestyle – parent, children very good, made life easier. Still taking drugs Class A B C. Now 8 years on morphine 35mg a day plus. Gave up all drugs except cannabis. Still riding motorcycles, fell in love with friend's wife! Oops! Susan.

1985

Married now with 5 children Nikki, Kai, Sarah, Clare, Andrew. Moved out of town into country village. Children grew, so did I. Good years fun and hard work.

Carol lost her life to cancer!

• 1990

Only child to loads of children, taught me so much.

Nikki left home to work and live with Paul. Kai moved out to live with Candice. Susan and I had fun, with less responsibilities, still travelling.

1995
Owned our house. Another new motorcycle, plus many
more runabouts. Sold house and moved back into town.
Andrew and Clare went to work. Began to travel again.
Various jobs, living pretty good. Susan diagnosed with
cancer. Mother died of cancer aged 66.
• **2000**
The millennium. Gave up work to look after Susan.
Lost house, Susan became ill, very. Susan and I travelled
constantly until her death on 5th of November 2003.
Now living in council flat. After Susan's death, went back to
Tunisia. December attacked in mountains near Algerian
border by four men. Badly injured but survived, luckily
carrying a knife.
2005
Injuries worsening already battered body.
2008
February, gave up riding motorcycles. Body failing.
Brain damaged, receptor areas. Spinal column collapsing,
chronic pain syndrome.
Started using wheelchair. Have own PA Andrea (carer).
2009
5th of November; 6 years now Susan died. Nearly at
the Finish Post! November travel back to Tunisia. Visit
my brother in Allah Jomma and family; now 16th visit!
Soon be Christmas, am disabled, slightly mad!
But I'm alive to tell you!
• **2010**
? The inner horizon, what lies beyond is already here.
60 plus.

Charlie Wolf's story
Excerpts from the Life Story of Charlie Wolf
*Charlie believes that he is suffering from PTSD (Post
Traumatic Stress Disorder), brought on by the sudden
and unexpected death of a young man in his home, as
described below in Part 2. Charlie is struggling to have
his diagnosis recognised by his doctor and specialist.
Charlie loves to write. Some of his life story is overleaf;*

his artwork is on the cover and his poem is in Chapter 5.

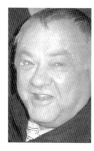

Part 1:

Born Graham Robert Burkmar, I was born on Shrubhill farm in Feltwell in northwest Norfolk, England. Feltwell is in the fenlands of Norfolk and anyone born in the fenlands of Norfolk is known as a 'fen tiger', whereas people born in other parts of Norfolk are called 'Norfolk Dumplings'. Graham was born on the 1st of March 1948: Saint David's Day (the patron saint of Wales). On Wood Farm where my father worked I got into some scrapes at three years old: once I was sat on the front of a stationary four wheel trailer behind a tractor. The tractor was being driven by Bob Cockerel. As Bob started to move I lost my balance and fell forward. According to what Bob told my parents I never yelled out but at the moment that I fell forward, in line with the big wheels, Bob turned around and saw me falling. He then stopped the tractor and picked me up. My Guardian Angel was looking out for me when Bob Cockerel turned around. Also on Wood Farm I climbed an oak tree and could not get down again. Another escapade was chasing bullocks with a stick. Once at the same tender age of three my father got me to steer the tractor while he forked out the hay to the cattle. So much for my adventures at three years old.

The next thing I remember is living in a caravan, still in Norfolk: I think I was approaching five years old but I did not go to school there. The most eventful thing that happened to me there was that while my mother was out one day I found a bar of chocolate: it was Exlax (a laxative). What a mess I was in later on: My mother was furious when she came home. We then left Norfolk and went to Hertfordshire, having sold the caravan I think. We lived near Hemel Hempstead on another farm. During that time I started school which was uneventful. I remember that my father was made temporary foreman for three months until they got a replacement for the one who had left. I remember feeling sorry for my father for not getting the job permanently as he was both good at his job and worked very hard. My mother worked as a nursing assistant in a mental hospital in St Albans in the nights and it used to scare her. I remember that when we lived there it was either bread and butter or bread and jam but not both.

Next stop was Dorset where we lived on a farm in a caravan. It was high up on the cliffs. It was near a village called Morecombelake. I remember that there were pigs on the farm from pictures that my parents kept. The nearest school was in Charmouth which was situated on the river Char. To get to school, we had to walk to Morecombelake and then catch a taxi all paid for by the local council.

I had a childhood sweetheart: her name was Roberta Dare. She later became a pathologist. Her father was a local farmer but they were very poor from what I can remember.I was only about seven years old then and I was already after the girls. The school at Charmouth was very strict and you were not allowed to interrupt the teacher for anything. I was bursting to go to the toilet big time and the teacher was in full flow. By the time I got up enough courage to interrupt him it was too late. It was the Exlax situation all over again. They got my coat and put it on me then called a taxi to take me home for my poor mother to clean up.

Part 2: *Here, Charlie describes in detail how his young friend died*
I rang the emergency doctor, Dr Connor, and he arrived at ten past five. He checked J.D. (pronounced 'jee day') a couple of times and at half past five he declared that he could not find anything wrong with him and yet I had told him over the phone that J.D. had abdominal pains, chest pains and was sweating profusely (symptoms which I later found out were classic text book symptoms of a dissecting aneurism). It had taken me three phone calls to convince him to come out in the first place: the first time he told me to put a hot water bottle on his stomach, the second time he told me to give him two Aspirins and the third time he

agreed to come out. When he left at half past five, he said to ring at half past eight if things were still the same and then one of them would come out and investigate further.

When I rang at half past eight and told him that J.D. was still the same he said that he was not going to abandon his surgery and that he would come out after eleven o'clock. Lill would not let me go to work because she knew that there was something seriously wrong. At two minutes past nine there was a loud groan from upstairs and when I rushed up I found J.D. collapsed on the floor. I thought he was messing around at first and then I realised that it was serious so I started to do mouth to mouth on him. I told Lill to ring for an ambulance and when she came back I got her to take over while I rang the doctor, telling him that the boy was dying. The truth was that he was dead. Both the doctor and the ambulance arrived and I went with the doctor and J.D. in the ambulance to the hospital, where he was declared dead at two minutes past ten.

I rang up work and my manager Larry Lowes came and gave me a lift back home and I was given a week's compassionate leave. During the following week, the French Embassy rang me up and gave me grief over the phone. Jean Michel and Annie came over from Paris for the funeral service, which was held at Reading Crematorium. They said that they wanted him to be cremated in Reading instead of Paris because he had been very happy with us in Reading. I bought a special funeral card and wrote my first poem in it. I put it on the dining room table where Jean Michel saw it and asked whether he could have it. During the funeral service I cried like I have never cried in my life. At the time I would have willingly changed places with J.D. if it had been possible. When I went back to work the only music that I listened to for the next six weeks was Mozart then all of a sudden I went back to the Rolling Stones, my favourite band.

After Jean Michel and Annie went back to Paris we received a copy of the coroner's report: there had been a post mortem because he was a foreign national and it was done by a Home Office Pathologist, with six police present because they thought it was suspicious circumstances. J.D. apparently had 'Marfans Syndrome', a rare condition where the skeletal growth takes off rapidly at puberty and anywhere between the ages of 9 and 65, the inner walls of the aorta weaken and rupture (a dissecting aneurism). Poor J.D.

Tina Lawlor Mottram's story
Balance, intuition and hope

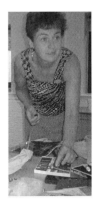

I guess my story began when I was 18 and a nurse handed me an orange and a syringe saying 'Practise on this. It's the closest to human skin.' I had spent months losing weight inexplicably; I was down to less than 7 stone from my normal weight of 9 and a half stone. I ate from morning to night, anything and everything in the house, anything extra going and still ravenously hungry. What I didn't realise was that my body was eating myself. Unable to digest food due to a lack of insulin, my body began to eat its fat reserves, until I looked like a famine victim. I was always so thirsty but I assumed everybody was like that. The tiredness I could explain away from late nights as a student. It wasn't until I started 'falling asleep' at college under tables that people started to notice. I was going into a hyperglycaemic coma. I was a diabetic.

Diabetes would have killed me a hundred years ago. Nowadays, it must be the only illness where you feel better immediately after you're diagnosed. The insulin injected means you feel energetic again for the first time in years and I actually gained a bit of weight. It was such a relief to be alive at all, that the restrictions of the condition hardly sank in. So you can't eat this, you can't eat that, you have to measure out your food in rations of carbohydrate and you see a specialist every month for a while. You have to test your urine every day and then test your blood.

Everybody talks about 'diabetic complications' in hushed tones and to be honest, you look at them like they're crazy. I'm only 18 I'm thinking. I'm not overweight, I don't smoke, I'm fit and I eat well. Often I look healthier than the doctors

I see. What are they on about? The realisation that actually you are ill and that you need to take care of yourself, for the rest of your life, dawns slowly. Balance is the key.

The group at work

Taking drugs long term is bad for the health, even if they're prescribed! Anybody knows that. Your blood sugars need to be between 4 and 7 on average. I have days when mine have been. Some days it works wonderfully. Other days it doesn't and I go hypo. I can't see the logical pattern in all this except that my body doesn't have the automatic 'shut off' insulin method that most people have, regulated by their own internal hormone system. My insulin is GM and factory manufactured. So when my blood sugar dips below 3 as it often does, I'm gasping for grub and groaning again.

Usually this occurs because I cycled too fast or did too much exercise at the allotment or a meal was delayed by 5 minutes or whatever. It is not easy to keep your blood sugar between 4 and 7, take it from me. Then your liver compensates. If you go hypo, it then releases stored energy, which means your blood sugars can register as high as 17 after a low. I've had to work hard at being healthy. I don't eat crap; I love fruit and veg. I have no car and get lots of exercise, both for health and environmental reasons. Balancing my need for some insulin with the exact amount of food I eat is what I keep getting wrong. I'd like to be put in touch with a diabetes specialist who isn't lecturing me about behaving badly. I'm not. It seems that if you are above a certain age and your Ha1C (blood test) isn't perfect, then they assume it's because you are eating the wrong things. I'm not.

I've had brilliant, interested diabetes specialists in my time so I have high standards. Dr McKenna in Dublin and Dr Lowy in Guy's hospital, for example. They used to look at my blood tests, tweak my insulin dosage and listen to my concerns. As a result, I was well controlled for years and I am the proud mother of a healthy daughter. Last year I met a specialist for the very first time at my annual appointment. "So you've been diabetic since you were 18? And no complications yet. Well, this is the start of it now." This reference was to a minute amount of blood found in my urine sample; which meant, according to her, that I was in the early stages of 'diabetic nephropathy', ie kidney failure to you and me.

Apparently this had been explained to me the previous year (says so in my notes) when I had been for my annual visit. I was open mouthed. I did not remember this; nor did I believe that her diagnosis was necessarily true. There are many reasons for blood in the urine, which need to be eliminated first. Apparently, I should have that test done soon but in the meantime, I should take this prescription: Ramipril. I come home convinced that I am at death's door. Tears, floods, internet research. I guess for the specialist, that means they recommended my taking these ace inhibitor drugs and that's them off the hook for litigation; it says so in the notes. When I get the drugs, I notice they are for high blood pressure.

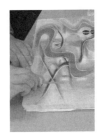

Tania's artwork can be seen in the Colour Section.

That's odd I think. I've always had really low blood pressure, sometimes almost abnormally so. I query this with my chemist; usually very knowledgeable. He thinks the drugs may offer some kidney protection but advises me to go back to check with my GP. I read the leaflet with Ramipril. "Do not take Ramipril if you have low blood pressure." Under side effects, I note that "Treatment with Ramipril may impair *renal* and liver function in some individuals." (italics are mine). The packet is still in my first aid cupboard, untouched almost a year later. Thank goodness, as time will tell.

It is a long wait to my next blood and urine tests, which will determine whether or not my kidneys are in trouble. I waited until I had the nerve to do a blood test about 8 months later. My results? I now have 'normal' kidney and liver function. And my PCR, used to examine my urine sample is also 'normal'. My GP says we won't change anything then. Good thing I didn't take the drugs? My GP says to discuss it with the specialist. After all, she prescribed them. I decide that I will. Maybe.

As I haven't seen my diabetes specialist for years because he saw me only when I first joined his clinic, from my point of view, there is no continuity of care, apart from Rachel, my diabetes nurse, who is wonderful. So I chat to her, we agree changes, and then learn to do it myself. I read, I research. Or I give up. Frequently I hover between both of these so I guess diabetes has taught me my life lesson: balance. I try. I really do. I eat well. I exercise. I don't smoke. I smile a lot. I argue my case with doctors. From my story, it is evident that I know my body *at least* as well as the specialists. More importantly, I know that I am on my body's side. It seems to me that presumptions are often made in the care of long term patients, like me.

Meditation helps me greatly and as I have a gift for healing, I've noticed that whenever I offer healing to anybody else, that seems to keep my blood sugars low too. The thing is, I take *only* my daily insulin injections. Nothing else. I get my vitamins from home grown organic allotment food, although I've been known to have a bottle of Rescue Remedy in my bag for emergencies. I don't want to be addicted to any new man-made drugs. My advice for anybody with a long term condition is that it's ok to have the odd bad day. Everybody does. Despite the illness, realising every single day at some stage that you are happy, alive and lucky is a recipe for good health and long life. It's worked for me up to now!

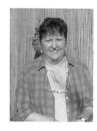

Rose Pope and her husband Raymond came to several sessions, having had the group recommended to her by the local hospital. Tania came along with Rose, both attending the same hospital for treatment. Rose and Tania quickly settled into painting, and Rose even offering Reiki healing from time to time. Unfortunately, Rose's time on the project was cut short, due to a fall in December and having to spend some time in hospital. Lynne found the group when we made a presentation to the Macmillan Coffee Morning in Chatham Library in 2009. She painted with the group, and tried some healing and meditation.

My idea in starting this group was to share some of the concerns you've read about in this first chapter with a group of other people who also have long term conditions. What was very lovely is that many people came along who were not themselves affected by illness but happy to take part as volunteers helping people to get to Sunlight or to the healing clinic. Some of those who care for those with illness, also enjoyed it very much. A few points about some of our concerns are listed below. If there are any medical professionals reading this and would like to get in touch, we'd love to hear from you.

• Prescriptions - am I getting the right drugs? It is difficult for many members of the group to collect prescriptions regularly. Is there a better way for people with long term conditions to get their medication? Are these new drugs you are prescribing addictive? Are there risks?

• Doctors need to listen to the 'experts' ie US. We know our bodies. Communication is always possible, if you try. If you don't believe in your doctor, switch.

• Misdiagnosis and/or sloppy diagnosis. Sarah, Charlie, Win and Tina have argued the case.

• Even if you are not 'ill', meditation helps. Ditto healing and deep breathing techniques. If you have got a long term condition, all of these are non invasive and worth a try. Even if you as a practitioner don't believe in these techniques, give them the benefit of the doubt. They don't harm the patient like addictive drugs. Perhaps doctors and nurses should be encouraged to have healing too, as is the case in UCLH[*3] in London, where Angie Buxton-King has brought healing into the NHS.

• Care gaps have been identified - transport, the weather eg getting to the chemist, the doctor, the hospital, taking the group to London; taxis to Sunlight. Public transport can be a nightmare if you are not 100%.

• Nobody should take away hope. There is always hope.

Doctors know that there are cases of inexplicable recoveries and miracles. So please don't deliver the results of tests in a really negative way. You can ruin a person's life for many months and years. If you give the diagnosis with kindness, then people will believe that you are a 'healer' doctor - one who tries to aid people, to help them cure, not plunge them into depression.

On a more positive note, everybody enjoys meeting at Sunlight, loves meditation and healing and most of us know we can paint now! Few of us want want to complain, despite not being taken seriously. We all want the best quality of life available, whatever our individual circumstances. What we all want and demand from our health care providers is information about our illnesses and then to take responsibility for it as much as we can. Finding the triggers, understanding how to keep healthy, accepting our limitations but never losing our spirit.

Now that the seeds of our stories have been planted, in the next few chapters, we will take you on our creative journey with all our illnesses throughout this year.

NOTES
[1] Roger Cook, The Tree of Life
[2] Dr Caroline Myss, Why people don't heal and how they can.
[3] University College London Hospital has employed healers Angie Buxton-King and Graham King to work in the hospital as paid members of staff and members of the multidisciplinary team. Now the hospital has a team of complementary therapists to offer to patients and their families.

Chapter 2
Spirituality, the afterlife and spiritual healing: a history

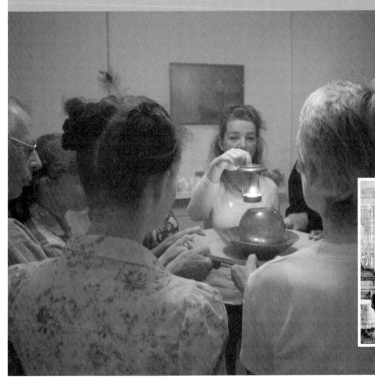

Meditation for healers in The Sanctuary prior to a day in the contact healing clinic in the College of Psychic Studies
Photo: Derek Wilkinson

Inset: Levitation by Daniel Dunglas Home, a college medium

There are more things in heaven and earth, Horatio, than are dreamt of in your philosophy.
Hamlet Act 1, Scene 5,
William Shakespeare

Energy cannot be created nor destroyed, merely tranformed.

The Oxford Concise Dictionary defines "health" as being *free of disease*. Marilyn Ferguson[1] concurs in 'The Aquarian Conspiracy' that as "we have defined health in negative terms, as the absence of disease, so we have defined peace as non-conflict. But peace is more fundamental than that." So, I would posit, is health. It is incredibly emotive; the group we recruited to look at illness creatively, are very conscious of levels of health – including feeling on top of the world, despite having a chronic long term condition, even if the medical experts do not agree that one is in good health. We can have a healthy appetite for life and we all know and quote the adage *healthy, wealthy and wise* and the old saying that *an apple a day keeps the doctor away*.

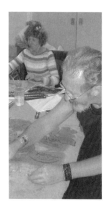

Lizz and Gordian daub paint on recycled sheets at a workshop at Sunlight in July 2009.

The word "spiritual" is taken from the Latin 'spiritus', meaning *breath of life*. Ask anybody what *spirit* is and the answers show the breadth of association in the human mind and vocabulary. It is somebody *spirited*, with a mischievous sense of fun and/or a strong opinion. *Spirit* is a cleanser, a solution of volatile compounds, like white spirit or turpentine. *Spirit* can be a person filled with the essence of the moment or a prevailing mood, as in 'the nation's egalitarian spirit'. It can take the form of a supernatural *spirit*, one who frequents dark spaces and lurks with a whiff of fear of the unknown (for some) and the embodiment of the essence of a person after death. *Spirit* can also be an alcoholic beverage; indeed many cultures have traditionally used stimulants, drugs and natural substances to reach a state of removal from the ordinary – the Maya for example, held ritual ceremonies associated with drinking large amounts of balché[2] an alcohol which enabled the drinkers to then speak to their ancestors and deities.

Balché was used ceremonially, to prepare individuals for certain religious rites and indeed to bestow god-like powers on the drinker. Trances induced by the drink (and perhaps by belief in its powers) supposedly provide those who imbibe with a glimpse into a sacred, invisible world. The shamanic liqueur is a mix of honey and water and the bark of the balché tree are added. The honey was also used medicinally, supposedly for gynaecological problems. The belief in spirits and ancestors was linked to the natural world; there were deities for unripe corn and ripe corn, the wind, flint, eagles, deer. Their calendendrical system had a name for each cycle, each linked to the World Tree[3] (for them the Ceiba tree) rooted in the Underworld, whose trunk widened in this world and its branches and leaves spanned the heavens and the spirit world. Dedicated priests and shamans in the culture could contact the spirit world, using ceremonies and blood sacrifice, often pictured in the stone carvings and the very rare manuscripts[4] which survived the Spanish invasion and plunder of the New World.

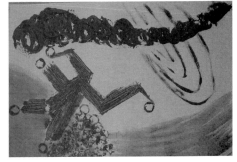

Artwork created on this project by Doug Fry The Wind. He identifies the wind as a natural force that can start the aches of Trigeminal Neuralgia.

Our creative group have shared many religious and spiritual and inexplicable experiences, which have taken place both at workshops and in their daily lives. Themes of death and illness have uncovered lost children, mothers, family members and spouses; many believe that they have had contact with their loved ones as they die, after their death, in their dreams and daydreams and in their own, everyday life. The belief in another world beyond this one runs through the fabric of almost every member of this group. For the author as a young child, an experience of death and the transition to another world began when she received a visit from her dying grandmother, who was in hospital in the last stages of terminal cancer.

I woke up in dead of night. We were all staying in my maternal gran's house and it was quite strange and eerie, partly because my family was in sleeping bags all over the floor. I felt obliged to nip past all of them, almost oblivious in dreamland, because although I couldn't see her, I could hear Gran talking to me. It wasn't like speaking; more a silent form of communication, which I now freely accept as an adult. I really wanted her to stay - we were talking about

55

gardening. She had given me my first trowel and fork. Gran had a gentle certainty that she was going and this was a goodbye, although reluctant from me. The next day, while we were driving to the hospital, me sitting squashed in the back of the car with my siblings, I recall wondering 'Why are we going? She's not there any more.' Then seeing my father come out of the hospital weeping, I simply kept my mouth shut. Years later, on revealing this to my uncle, he revealed that Gran had also visited him at work that night. He was a journalist, used to working night shifts, perhaps night time being more conducive to visits from the other side!

For some members of this group, deep spirituality is embodied in their faith and in their church, like Gill, Derrick and James who run a group for people with Cerebellar Ataxia.[5] Gill's group helps people to come to terms with their rare disease and comforts them with a home cooked meal once a month, a social exchange and a chance to talk to people who really understand. Gill's lifetime has been one of living with a condition that makes being *alive* a gift. She was not expected to live in her childhood and was also told that she would never have children. She is still very much alive and has 3 children. Gill's Nan, Constance, and her husband Jim brought up the family, after Gill's mother had died in childbirth. Gill recalls being bullied very badly at school due to her physcial disabilities and being unable to do PE. Coming home one day battered, bruised and in tears, Constance sat her down and gave her a pep talk about life.

"Nan said come here, I'm going to wash those tears" recalls Gill. "She's the bully, she's got the problem, not you. She has to live with her conscience. Turn it around. Take what you've learned and help somebody else. You'll live." It was very good advice Gill recognises, even now, and she has lived this line all her life. Gill nursed Constance who died aged 81; however, Nan still comes to her in times of great need "She came to me at times because I couldn't cope" said Gill. I can't imagine Gill not coping. She has the quiet determination to live every day as it if were her last, helping with a kind word and her enthusiasm, despite all the difficulties life has thrown at her. Her ability to 'turn it round' is remarkable.

For other members of our group, their quiet faith in the spiritual and the intuition, comes with or without a religion; for most, it is a heart-held belief that their loved ones are still in some way, with them; looking after them, guiding them and loving them. Gordian's story is losing not one, but two wives, and he recounts sitting in spiritualist churches after the death of Susan, his second wife, at the back, simply not wanting to hear. Nevertheless, on one occasion he was selected by a medium, who wanted to give him a message, which made sense. I must also thank Gordian for lending me his very beloved, ancient, valuable copy of "The Blue Island" by William Thomas Stead.

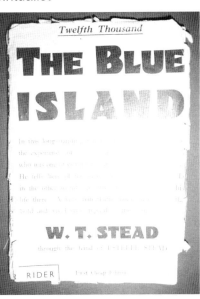

As I read, I feel that I am handling a piece of history itself; the cover is falling off and I resist my urge to tape it back on. If this were my book, I tell myself, I would patch it up and have it rebound, but as I am in fear of damaging a loan from a now very dear friend, I am simply grateful. As I read, I handle it with the utmost care, absorbing its message. It is an account of a journalist who was lost on board the ill-fated Titanic, whose spirit returned to write the book as recorded by a medium, Pardoe Woodman and Estelle Stead, his daughter. It starts with the letter of introduction[6] from Sir Arthur Conan Doyle, author of detective Sherlock Holmes and President of the College of Psychic Studies in the 1920s, who had a keen interest in the occult. He became fascinated by "life beyond the veil" particularly after losing his first wife Louisa. When he joined the Society for Psychical Research, it was considered to be a public declaration of his interest and belief in the occult. As Sherlock Holmes

Front cover of 'The Blue Island' by W T Stead Courtesy of Gordian Bailey

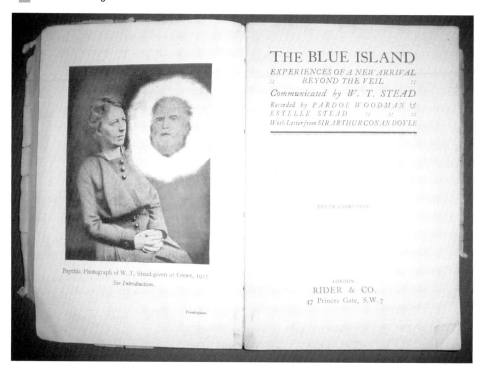

THE BLUE ISLAND

EXPERIENCES OF A NEW ARRIVAL
:: *BEYOND THE VEIL* ::

Communicated by W. T. STEAD

Recorded by PARDOE WOODMAN &
ESTELLE STEAD :: ::
With Letter from SIR ARTHUR CONAN DOYLE

Psychic Photograph of W. T. Stead given at Crewe, 1915
See Introduction.

LONDON
RIDER & CO.
47 Princes Gate, S.W.7

Above:
Frontispiece of 'The Blue Island' with Stead's psychic photograph with his daughter.

said to Watson, "Work is the best antidote to sorrow…" Starting with this introduction as a taster of the quirks of the supernatural, I race through the book in one sitting.

The frontispiece,[7] with Stead's face (see above) is a "psychic photograph" beside his daughter Estelle, given at Crewe in 1915, which leaves me interested and also aware that at one stage in my life I would have been sceptical, wondering if this were a fake, mainly because I would not know how this photograph could have been made. The whole process is described in detail in the book and since 1912 was hardly the days of Photoshop editing, I begin to read and try to understand how this book came to light. The words speak for themselves.

As I read their beauty reaches me. A series of events in my own life have led to my certainty that spirit exists, all around us, and in our daily existance if we allow the wisdom to come. It is as elusive as can be, because our minds cannot use even 20% of their potential. However, this is a journey made by every individual and I can never make it for anybody else. These words of William Thomas Stead speak for themselves. The description of the world (and perhaps worlds) after this one, are so tangible and they feel so right in a gut instinct manner, that for me it simply makes sense to read it, then accept the wisdom and the importance of his message.

William Thomas Stead was one of the most controversial men of his age. The most famous passenger aboard the ill-fated Titanic, he had a greater measure of notoriety than most British statesmen. As a journalist and editor, he was an important contributor to the birth of today's powerful tabloid journalism, and as a spiritualist and pacifist, his many social and spiritual campaigns had far reaching effects that remain with us today. Yet, posterity barely remembers him, except as an obscure figure in the hinterland of journalistic history. His book is serene; attempting to convey to us the essence of life after death.

Below: The author in life: W T Stead. Photos courtesy of W.T. Stead Resource Site

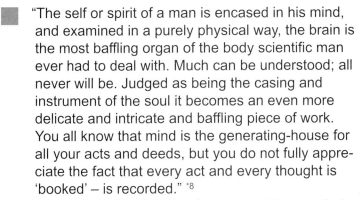 "The self or spirit of a man is encased in his mind, and examined in a purely physical way, the brain is the most baffling organ of the body scientific man ever had to deal with. Much can be understood; all never will be. Judged as being the casing and instrument of the soul it becomes an even more delicate and intricate and baffling piece of work. You all know that mind is the generating-house for all your acts and deeds, but you do not fully appreciate the fact that every act and every thought is 'booked' – is recorded." [*8]

The message of the book for me is one we all know; that "if people on earth realised the result of their thoughts upon those to whom they refer, they would be very much more careful in giving their mind free play. There are so many thoughts possible, and all of them registered here; many of them affect the people they concern, but all of them affect the people from whom they emanate." He reiterates the idea by saying that we are fully aware of the influence given out by any one person who is deeply depressed or more than usually excited or happy. His belief is that these are caused by lowered or raised mental vibrations. He continues: "That is why I say that whilst on earth it is not only advisable, but essential to keep your minds under control and in order. It is only wisdom to do so. The difficulty is that people will not realise this whilst upon earth, although they know from their own inner consciousness that I am stating a truth. I want you all to realise the results you are making, the unhappiness you are causing others, and the regret and sorrow you are laying up for yourselves in the next world when you have to face the conditions you have made. Remember that your minds are the generating-houses. You are building up whatever is to be your next condition, precisely and by the degree to which your body controls your mind instead of the mind ruling supreme."

Arthur Conan Doyle wrote the introduction to The Blue Island

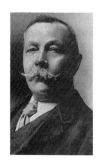

Sir Conan Doyle's great experience into research about the afterlife is referred to in the introduction, stating that he can hardly think of anyone has read more accounts, printed, typed and written, than he has done. He points out that this blue island is not specifically mentioned in any other manuscript. However, he agrees that in any event there are hardly 2 witnesses who would agree on all details even in this world and also maintained that "the colour blue is of course, that of healing, and an island may be only an isolated sphere – the ante-chamber to others."

Spirituality and belief in another world after this one allow people to live lives here with much more peace. Most (complementary) practitioners share an underlying belief that mind, body and spirit are connected. Health is a state of harmony and balance among the forces - energies, gods, or spirits – thought to govern the whole being. Sickness is a contrary state of disease or conflict among those forces. The idea is hardly unique to this century; it recalls millenniums old Chinese, Indian and very ancient worldwide traditions that simply imply the same conclusion; all ailments, from the common cold to cancer, are symptoms of more profound disruptions in the inner being.

Perhaps the roots of healing and ancient medicine can be seen in ancient cave paintings and the remaining artifacts from both Africa and Siberia, the roots of trance healing. Some of ancient therapies go back perhaps 40,000 years to the healer-priests who served the tribes of ancient Stone Age hunter gatherers, known as shamans. This term, that originated with North Asian, Ural Altaic, and Paleoasian peoples, is still widely used. Modern ethnology studies of the shaman in the ancient arts and traditions of America, Central Asia, Africa and South East India and Australia provide clues to ancient cultures, mysteries and healing medicine.

Nepalese shamans have been observed in modern times in trance, chanting mantras, and using grains of rice on a ceremonial plate to divine the nature of the illness. In Tibet, dancing using streamers is a common practice. Many observers have seen some stamp on hot coals in bare feet and emerge unscathed. In Egypt, ancient papyri reveal that incantations and medications varied from disease to disease and shamans often recommended the wearing of an amulet to cure the patient. Advice was offered in the form of herbs, meditation, fasting, prayers, songs and chants. Shamans do not normally choose their vocation; they are often called to it in a very powerful way. This can take place by having an illness themselves, by a powerful dream, a meeting with a teacher, a vision quest. The shaman[9] may ascend the 'world-tree' and by some method, sometimes with a guide, pass into the celestial realm. Shamans traditionally work mainly at night, by firelight, and often in a place designated as sacred – for example, a cave, a mountain top, close to a spring, where healing energy will be most vibrant. The shaman's 'rite of passage' is often a public ceremony but is sometimes associated with a symbolic death and resurrection or transformation. In the Christian faith, Saint Paul had a conversion en route to Damascus, which is discussed in Ray Brown's story later in this chapter.

Humanity has integrated the idea of spirituality, both consciously and unconsciously for centuries. Carlos

Castaneda experimented with hallucinative drugs and herbs including peyote, with his mentor Don Juan. 'The Teachings of Don Juan' in 1968, was the first in a series of books that describe Castaneda's training in traditional Mesoamerican shamanism. His books have sold more than 8 million copies in 17 languages. Castaneda's books are in the first person as an account of the author's meeting with a shaman and his experiences using hallinatory drugs and the lessons he learned. Some critics label them as works of fiction, attacking the author's lack of data and evidence. For me, they are valuable insights and like 'The Blue Island', a compelling read, whose truth seems to resound within me. Stories hold truths for me, be they ancient myths and fairytales or modern paperbacks and I am certainly a fan! Concepts such as time and 'reality' are explored in ways which the author labelled as 'nonordinary reality.' It is all too easy to dismiss a concept because it is not fully understood.

Maxwell Cade [10] (see Chapter 4) explored states of consciousness ranging from Level 0 (sleep), Level 1 (dreaming sleep) and up to 8 levels labelled from 'waking sleep' through to 'cosmic consciousness unity' in his Level 8. Mystical states are described by religions and believers worldwide, in addition to many scientists, philosophers writers and creatives including Maharishi, Gurdjieff, Wallace, Maslow, and Jung among many.

Ayahuasca was explored as a treatment for a medical diagnosis by Donald M. Topping[11], Ph.D. Professor Emeritus, University of Hawaii President, Drug Policy Forum of Hawaii, who encouraged western physicians to "take the drug as a serious tool to cure ill health." Jeremy Narby, was intrigued by claims by Peruvian Indians that their knowlege of medicinal plants and biochemistry had been communicated to them while under the influence of hallucinogens. In 'The Cosmic Serpent' Narby quotes research by Luna[12] (1984), in which spirits present themselves during dreams and visions; showing how to diagnose illness, which plants to use and how, how to suck out the illness or restore the spirit to a patient.

The 1960s saw an explosion in the use of LSD and other psychedelic drugs, to achieve a similar effect. However, mankind has used other, less damaging ways for the body to reach this state of other worldliness. Meditation is one and this practice is widespread across the globe; using breath control the body can convert its mind waves from everyday 'beta' waves to the more dreamlike ones typical of altered consciousness such as theta, delta and alpha waves. See Chapter 4 for more details of brain patterns recorded during meditation; and more information about auras and research.

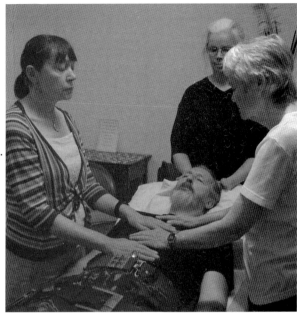

Gordian from our creative group, who visited the group healing clinic in the College of Psychic Studies in July 2009. Shown with Cynthia (left), Kathy and June (right) in The Sanctuary.
Photo: Derek Wilkinson

Dr Daniel J Benor in 'Spiritual Healing' writes that "the mechanical and biochemical models" favoured by conventional medicine cannot explain many aspects of health and illness. The mind and body are intimately linked, each influencing the other eg hypnotic and post anaesthetic suggestion can dramatically alleviate pain and other post-surgical discomforts and complications."[*13]

Dr Daniel J Benor has compiled research papers from recognised institutions all over the world, in an effort to validate the work of spiritual healing, combined with conventional medicine and psychotherapy. In a personal communication in December 2009, Dr Benor[*13] agrees that conventional medicine "is most helpful in treating infections, physical trauma, and hormonal problems and helpful in providing systematized diagnoses." Being particularly interested in the case of people with long term conditions, such as our group, he commented that conventional medicine "is very limited and often creates more problems when dealing with chronic illnesses, because it is limited to medication interventions that carry serious side effects. In the US alone, over 100,000 people die every year from negative effects of medications properly prescribed, and another 150,000 from medical errors and complications. This makes conventional medicine the third leading cause of death, after cancer and heart disease. You are more likely to die from medical care than from motor vehicle accidents or violent crimes or accidents in your home!"

Dr Benor continues that spiritual healing can contribute significantly to treatment of long-term care in many ways, such as alleviation of pain and stress reactions, decreases in severity of physical and psychological symptoms, and in some cases with cures of diseases. "My own area of interest has been in the felicitous combination of spiritual healing with psychotherapy, where each modality again nicely complements the other. Spiritual healing often brings about releases of emotions that were long buried, which can be processed in psychotherapy. Psychotherapy raises buried feelings that may be troublesome and often encounters blocks to progress that can be helped by spiritual healing."

Scientific medicine has sometimes taken a dim view of 'complementary' approaches to health and healing, despite their existence for many centuries in most cultures worldwide. Since the 18th century in Europe, medicine has been in the hands of the scientists, some of whom have viewed the body almost as mechanical, supplying tests for this and drugs for that and often accused of merely dealing with the symptoms by the patient. As complementary care views the person with mind, body and spirit interlinked, health is a state of harmony and balance in the whole body, including mind and spirit. Therapists work to the idea that if one of these is out of balance, then disease may occur. Much of this type of care can be preventative and effective breathing techniques alone can often be a first step to better health...

When one's body does go out of balance, often the news is broken by the results of a diagnostic test at a GP surgery or hospital. The lack of hope offered by her diagnosis sent one of our group, Sarah, in search of more information, unable to accept the label given by medicine. Other members of the group share her concern. Win remains convinced that her son could have been saved. The author spent almost a year of her life worrying that she had diabetic nephropathy, after a consultant she had met just once stated that it was so. In fact, further tests and the patient's own intuition about her body proved correct and the next blood samples showed normal kidney function. However, the time in-between was like a death sentence at times. Stuck between wanting to do the the test to confirm or not, yet too scared to actually take the test and the underlying effect of this on this family's life was fairly horrendous. As well as totally unnecessary.

Dr Bernie Siegel, who works with groups of cancer patients in his ECaP[*14] programme, is adamant that there is a need for optimism when giving a diagnosis. The truth can always be delivered 'with hope' he says, because who really knows what the future will bring? Often when faced with a diagnosis which seems to lack hope from doctors, this is a time when people reach for complementary treatments such as healing. This book looks at spiritual healing in the sense of a natural energy therapy with no invasive nor harmful side effects, which treats the whole person – mind, body and spirit. David Furlong[*15] writes in 'The Complete Healer' that it was realised in many esoteric traditions that the universe was held together by certain principle energies. He states that science is aware of many of these forces at a physical level, but there are many spectrums beyond dense matter. These powers permeate the collective unconscious of humanity. In order to make them more real and comprehend their quality, Furlong maintains that most cultures have designated their characteristics to different gods and goddesses.

In Taoist belief, these principles are reflected in the 8 trigrams of the I Ching[*16] an ancient divinatory tradition from China, known as The Book of Change. Used by the Chinese and many Western scholars, it is tradtionally used for determining the answer to a question about one's life. The I Ching was frequently used by Carl Gustav Jung, whose work on archetypes and the collective unconscious is well known. The 8 trigrams which are the basic building blocks of the system, (see left) consist of broken and unbroken lines, which are drawn from natural forces - heaven (sky), earth, mountain, water, wind, fire, thunder and lake. In Christianity these universal principles have been grafted on to key personages of the Christian story as well as the archangels, like Raphael and Gabriel. Furlong[14] maintains that by reading across mythologies we can gain an amazing insight into the working of these forces, using the colour spectrum as a model.

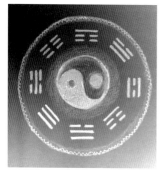

Bagua wheel of the I Ching
Tina Lawlor Mottram

Imagine the generative force of the universe, whether we call this God, Allah or whatever, as a white light. This moves out from the source and hits the spectrum of the cosmos, so splitting into a myriad of colours. Certain patterns of this energy have been more dominant in the formation of planet earth and Furlong maintains that the spiritual leaders of all cultures have appreciated this. This is why when we examine all the major religions, there is a very similar message to be found.

Healing; a brief history

Every country has its own laws regarding those who practise medicine and also those who work in healing. One of the most famous healers must surely be Jesus Christ, who reputedly cured the sick by the laying on of hands. Lepers, cripples, the lame and even the dead, responded to his healing touch. The Bible has many accounts of miraculous healings, merely by touching his clothes. Jesus said that "He that believes in me will also do the works I do… Whatever you ask in my name, I will do it." (John 14:12-13) The Church followed his lead in healing for many years after his death, in the tradition laid down by Jesus. He had commanded his disciples to preach the gospel and to heal the sick. From the Middle Ages, healing became a maverick art and in the 20th century, some churches still warned that those who practised it without its sanction were guilty of witchcraft or of being in league with the devil. For healers practising in the UK today, it is often the case that there is disbelief, derision and other responses by people who come to their first session, convinced that it will do them no good.

In ancient Greece, the equivalent of the shaman healer existed in the form of healing gods and deities. Asclepius (Latin Aesculapius) is the god of medicine and healing in ancient Greek religion. The son of Apollo, his mother was killed for being unfaithful to the god, but the unborn child was rescued from her womb. From this he received the name Asclepius meaning *to cut open*. Apollo carried the baby to the centaur Chiron, who raised Asclepius and instructed him in the art of medicine.

The rod of Asclepius, a snake-entwined staff, remains a symbol of medicine today. The snake is seen in many cultures as a creature of transformation and rebirth, due to the way it sheds its skin. Snakes were often used in healing rituals and non-venomous snakes were allowed to crawl on the floor in dormitories where the sick and injured slept. Asclepius' skills as a healer were almost too miraculous and after bringing people back to life from the dead, it is said that Hades thought that no more dead spirits would come to the Underworld, and so asked his brother to remove him. This angered Apollo who in turn murdered the cyclops who made the thunderbolt for Zeus. For this act, Zeus banned Apollo from the night sky and commanded Apollo to serve Admetus, King of Thessaly. After Asclepius' death, Zeus placed Asclepius among the stars as the constellation Ophiuchus ("the Serpent Holder"). Many temples of Asclepius were located all over Greece, including one on the island of Kos, where Hippocrates may have started his career. Hippocrates' name was part of the original doctor's permission to practise (in their Hippocratic Oath). In honor of Asclepius, from about 300 BC, the cult

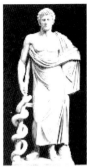

Asclepius, Greek god of medicine and healing, with his snake entwined rod, widely used as a symbol of medicine, even in modern times. *Photo / Citation Wikipedia, The Free Encyclopedia* *17

of Asclepius grew very popular and pilgrims flocked to his healing temples (Asclepieia) to be cured of their ills. Often the patient would stay the night in these sanctuaries and dream interpretation would take place, which would offer them hope of curing their illnesses.

From The King's Touch to the modern day
In England and France, *The King's Touch* was well known as a way to cure sickness and this tradition was continued in England until the time of the Civil War. Valentine Greatrakes, who was born in 1628, was brought up in the Puritan tradition and he fought for Cromwell in the Civil War as a cavalry lieutenant in Waterford in Ireland. He was a wealthy, well respected man who was made a High Sheriff of Waterford in 1666. Although a very respectable member of society, Greatrakes discovered an unusual talent when he was 34; what he described as an impulse or *strange persuasion*'[18] This was his power to heal "The King's Evil" ie scrofula, a disease which disfigures the face and the body. During the 17th century it was widespread among the population in the UK and Ireland and with no monarch, Greatrakes felt able to provide his healing touch to those who needed it. In the UK in the 21st century, healers are able to practise openly, while in many countries at the time of writing, the practice of healing is illegal. Most European countries ban 'fringe' therapies and a case in Germany in 1981 led to the arrest and prosecution of healer, Josef Muller, for healing a sports wound of well known athlete Jo Deckarm in a hospital.

While interviewing healer Ray Brown'[19] and his spirit doctor Paul, he reminded me that until fairly recently in the Channel Islands, healers could still be prosecuted under witchcraft laws. Ray Brown has also faced problems with various national bodies of healers, for healing while being filmed, while in trance. Healer Harry Edwards struggled in vain to have healers admitted to hospitals. Angie Buxton King and Graham King are both now working as healers in the NHS in the UK and running courses for healers to enable them to do so - see later in this chapter.

The Chakra System

Those trained and accredited as healers in the College of Psychic Studies (and elsewhere) work with connecting to universal love and light and energy, channelled through the healer's hands and in contact healing, aimed at balancing the *chakra* system. The concept of the *chakra* is an integral part of Hindu and Yogic tradition.

The word "Chakra" comes from Sanskrit, where it literally means 'a wheel'. The word *chakra* also carries an implication of movement, so a more exact translation would be 'a moving wheel' or 'spinning wheel'. These centres in the body, located at the crown of the head, the brow, the throat, the heart, the solar plexus, the abdomen and the base of the spine are used as key balancing points within us.

Early research on the *chakra* energy system was carried out by CW Leadbeater from the Theosophical Society. More recently, the *chakras* have become associated with a rainbow of colours, starting with violet at the crown and descending through the rainbow colours - indigo at the brow, blue at the throat and so on to the red of the base *chakra* at the end of the spine.

However, Furlong[15] adds that this colour association with the spectrum is a recent addition to chakric knowledge. Nor was it confirmed by the early research work on chakras carried out by CW Leadbeater from the Theosophical Society. His research showed that green was linked with the solar plexus centre and gold with the heart.

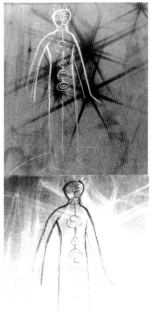

The chakra system, a series of illustrations by Tina Lawlor Mottram

Franz Anton Mesmer

He was born in 1733 in Austria; he graduated in medicine in Vienna in 1764. In 1766 he was studying what he called 'animal magnetism', which later became known as 'mesmerism'. He claimed this was a force which existed everywhere, most concentrated in magnets. His methods and treatments were famous and theatrical – in dim light, people were immersed in large wooden tubs, in which he placed glass bottles filled with iron filings and iron rods protruding from the tubs. Music was also played, which added to the sense of theatre. Mesmer himself would place himself close to the patients in the tub, holding an iron wand, which touched the affected area of the person. Treatments could last for hours and those in the tubs had Mesmer, dressed extravagantly in exotic clothes, staring at them; maybe stroking their ailing leg (or whatever part of the body was in need of treatment). *Mesmerists*, those who used his method, believed that blood was affected by magnets. After many hours, people began to choke, have fits, involuntary jerking movements, rolling eyes and this was known as the *crisis*, which preceded relief from their complaints. Mesmer had discovered there is an electro-magnetic force that emanates from us, which can be used to help others. Nowadays we call this the *aura,* which will be discussed in detail in Chapter 4.

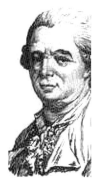

Above; Franz Anton Mesmer

Edgar Cayce

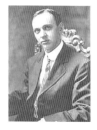

Below; Edgar Cayce in 1910

Edgar Cayce (1877-1945) has been called the "sleeping prophet" due to his psychic readings given while in trance, diagnosing illnesses and revealing lives lived in the past and prophecies yet to come. Cayce was born on a farm in Kentucky in the US in 1877. He showed some psychic abilities in childhood, and often played with "imaginary friends" whom he said were spirits on the other side. He also displayed an uncanny ability to memorize the pages of a book, simply by sleeping on it. However, it was not until the age of 16, when Cayce was struck by a ball at the base of his spine during a sports event, that his special abilities began to show. He wasn't seriously injured at the time, he seemed able to walk and converse; however, during that evening, he began to shout and roar at his family, in a manner quite unlike their boy. His family sent him to bed, where the boy fell into a deep sleep. While his parents watched over him, a strange voice (seemingly coming from Edgar) suddenly announced that Mrs Cayce should prepare a special poultice and lay it on the back of

his head. She followed the instructions from the mysteri-
ous voice and Edgar woke the next morning with no
memory of all that had passed the day or night before.

Afterwards, Cayce continued at school, then found
employment, but was forced to give up work because of
a series of severe headaches and sore throats. He tried
many treatments from physicians but none was able to
cure him. In desperation, after a year of putting up with his
headaches, Cayce turned to a local hypnotist Al Layne.
Cayce was reluctant to be hypnotised; rather he wanted
the hypnotist to act as his conductor once trance was
established. Cayce was instructed by Layne to look at his
body, locate the trouble and describe what he saw.

Then Cayce mumbled some words that would become
his trademark for many years to come. "Yes, we can see
the body." Cayce then announced that his problems lay in
his neck were because of partial paralysis of the vocal
cords. Layne asked him to increase blood circulation to his
throat by means of hypnotic suggestion. "His throat flushed
a violent red for 20 minutes, then he woke up, spat out
some blood and declared himself cured."[*20] After this, he
spent 40 years as "The Sleeping Prophet", devoting his life
to healing, psychic readings and dream interpretations.

He used to go into trance twice daily with his wife,
Gertrude, taking notes. Often clients visited him in person
but as his fame grew, he received many letters requesting
his help. Although unknown to him, these names and
addresses would be read to Cayce while in trance, and
he claimed that he could 'see' the body. He went on to
diagnose the illness of the named person and supplied a
list of recommendations for healing.

Edgar Cayce was a devoted churchgoer and Sunday
school teacher. At a young age, Cayce vowed to read the
Bible for every year of his life, and at the time of his death
in 1945, he had accomplished this task. He died in 1945,
leaving behind the Association for Research and
Enlightenment. His responses to questions he was asked
came to be called "readings" and their insights offer
practical help and advice to individuals even today.

Cayce's readings include 10,000 different topics including:
• Health-Related Information
• Philosophy and Reincarnation
• Dreams and Dream Interpretation
• ESP and Psychic Phenomena
• Spiritual Growth, Meditation and Prayer

Later in life, Cayce would find that he had the ability to put himself into a sleep-like state by lying down on a couch, closing his eyes, and folding his hands over his stomach. In this state of relaxation and meditation, he was able to place his mind in contact with all time and space — the universal consciousness, also known as the super-conscious mind. The majority of Edgar Cayce's readings deal with holistic health and the treatment of illness. Yet, although best known for this material, the sleeping Cayce did not seem to be limited to concerns about the physical body. Perhaps the readings said it best. When asked how to become more psychic, Cayce's advice was to become more spiritual.

Dorothy Kerin (1889 - 1963)

Dorothy Kerin
Photo courtesy of
Burrswood
Hospital and
Place of Healing

In 1912 Dorothy Kerin was a 22 year-old, who had been had been confined to bed for five years with tubercular meningitis, peritonitis and diabetes. Severe haemorrages had been frequent and many times doctors had predicted her death. Overnight, a miraculous cure restored her to full health; she and her sister heard beautiful voices singing and she saw a golden light while taking Holy Communion. Some of the spirit presences she described carried lilies and flowers. Much to the amazement of her family, she heard a voice saying "Dorothy your sufferings are over. Get up and walk." A full recovery took place. Her healing earned her national attention and press headlines of 'Miracle Girl'. Her physician Dr Norman was called and he was delighted with her recovery. He made a statement in the 'Daily Chronicle' (February 22nd, 1912) saying he had no idea how she had recovered and she had suffered enough to kill 5 people.[*21]

Kerin's personal experience was embodied in the idea

of the living Christ turning her life around - literally taking her from death to healthy life in a moment – and her life's mission became to provide a place where others could come to find the same healing from God, which she believed she had herself received. Kerin successively established three homes of prayer and healing in southern England from 1929 onwards. She believed she had a commission from God to 'heal the sick, comfort the sorrowing and give faith to the faithless.'

Burrswood was founded in 1948 after the war, when she moved to Speldhurst in Kent, and she purchased the land and buildings making up the core of the present-day Burrswood estate. All the funding and financial support came, as it had done in London, from donations. Dorothy Kerin pioneered what is now generally termed 'whole-person care', that is, she understood that physical illness cannot be separated from a person's spiritual, mental or emotional state, and that people must be cared for as a whole – body, mind and spirit. She firmly believed in bringing together mainstream medicine and Christian healing, and from the beginning she worked closely with the local vicar and GP to look after those entrusted to her care. For the rest of her life, she relied on the skills of trained professionals, and Burrswood became a fully -registered hospital in 2000.

Throughout her life, Kerin attracted a widespread following – and some measure of controversy – for her pioneering work in Christian healing. In later years, she drew worldwide support and praise from, among others, the then Archbishop of Canterbury, Dr Cosmo Lang and the American evangelist, Dr Norman Vincent Peale. The present Archbishop of Canterbury, Dr Rowan Williams is now a Patron of Burrswood, and the work of Burrswood is supported by the Church of England; as it is by the many healthcare professionals who refer their patients to it.

George Chapman and Dr Lang (1921–2006)

George Chapman was a trance healer and medium. Active for 60 years, Chapman treated patients by going into a state of trance and allowing the spirit of medical doctor William Lang to "operate" through him. He treated patients from all walks of life, including celebrities and members of the medical profession. After leaving school he was a garage hand, butcher and docker before becoming a professional boxer, later joining the Irish Guards in 1939. Chapman was transferred to the Royal Air Force as a gunner. After leaving the forces, he joined the fire brigade. He met and married Margaret May Dickinson in 1944. The Chapmans were devastated by the death of their first child Vivian in 1945, who survived only four weeks. When they used a glass-and-alphabet system, they received spirit messages telling them their daughter was alive and well in the next world. These experiments also induced a trance state in Chapman, and a variety of "entities" spoke through him. In time, however, "Dr Lang" manifested himself, explaining that his mission was to heal the sick.

William Lang, the son of a wealthy merchant, had been an ophthalmic surgeon at London's Middlesex Hospital from 1880 to 1914 and "operated" through Chapman. The age difference was that the surgeon would have retired from medical practice when Chapman was in his teens. Over the years many celebrities visited Chapman, including Laurence Harvey, Stanley Holloway, Patricia Neal, Barbara Cartland and Roald Dahl. Chapman's "surgery" on his patients was carried out on their spirit (or etheric) bodies, from which the benefits were transferred to the subjects' physical bodies. Among other cancers, he was credited with curing an inoperable and malignant brain tumour, as well as with improving various eye conditions and even lengthening a patient's leg. 'The Return of William Lang' was written about his life by S.G. Miron, whose wife was healed by Chapman with Lang's intervention. William Lang's daughter, Lyndon, and his grand-daughter, Susan Fairtlough, confirmed not only that his speech and mannerisms were as they remembered them, but also that they discussed events and people who would have been unknown to Chapman, who was not even in his teens when Lang retired from private medical practice. His cultured tones from beyond the grave were a stark contrast to those of the Liverpudlian fireman through whom he spoke. Lyndon Lang was so impressed with Chapman's mediumship that she contracted him to hold bi-monthly meetings at her home in London, for her friends and medical contemporaries of her brother, Basil Lang (also a surgeon), most of whom had known William Lang. This arrangement continued for ten years while Chapman continued to serve as a fireman and also held healing clinics, mostly in the Midlands.

Chapman left the fire brigade in 1956 which gave him more time to see patients and to travel. Eventually, he ran regular clinics in Paris and Lausanne, and carried out spirit operations in the United States, Canada, India and elsewhere. Lyndon Lang showed her support for Chapman and his mediumship by leaving much of her estate to him on her death in May 1977. By then, Chapman had moved to Pant Glas, close to Machynlleth, Wales. A healing clinic adjoined the house, where the medium slept in William Lang's bed, a gift from the surgeon's daughter.

Chapman himself always maintained that the purpose of his healing mission was to prove that there was life after death; he said the healings were secondary. This feeling was shared with many other healers including Cayce and Edwards and spiritualists, both in the past and the present.

Rose Gladden

Rose Gladden was the healer who worked with Andrew Buchan in 1969. The boy had an inoperable brain tumour, which led to him being confined to a wheelchair and his local football team, the Luton Town Players invited him to watch them play a match. One of the team members asked Andrew's family if they had ever considered spiritual healing. They never had, but they took him to see Rose Gladden and within five weeks, he was making a dramatic recovery. The doctor at the hospital was delighted and confused. "Andrew's recovery is truly amazing" was the headline in an article in 'Fate'in November 1978.

Rose Gladden was also one of the healers with whom Maxwell Cade worked during his research project funded by the Oliver Fisher Award from the College of Psychic studies in 1975 and 76. Cade explored Biofeedback and his 'Mind Mirror'; the science of listening to the body and using the results to help the mind to control the body. His book with Nona Coxhead entitled 'The Awakened Mind' is a must for anybody looking for interesting research about the effects of meditation and healing and scientific feed-back about how these processes affect the human body. It is available to borrow from the College of Psychic Studies library and it boasts a signed message by the author.

Below:
Rose Gladden
Photo courtesy
of Lindy Cowling

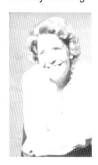

One of the highlights of these research experiments with healers and the 'Mind Mirror' took place at the Wrekin Trust Annual Conference at Loughborough in 1977.'[22] Healer Rose Gladden had agreed to demonstrate "fifth-state healing" before an audience. The audience on this occasion was comprised of 400 doctors, scientists, psychologists, healers and lay people and the whole event was televised. Norah Forbes had volunteered to act as a subject for a demonstration by Maxwell Cade to show the synchronicity of brain wave patterns that occurs when a healer treats a patient. Gladden described for the group her way of attuning to he healing energy. It had unshake-able patterns, that could be shown on the Mind Mirror, in front of hundreds of people or before television cameras. Rose described her method of 'attunement' in David Harvey's 'The Power to Heal'.'[23] "You attune yourself to a level where there is tremendous power and love." Rose also said she needed to attune to the person to whom the healing was sent. Max Cade had wired up both the healer and the healee to Mind Mirrors portable EEG (electro-encephalograph) machines.

Forbes describes her experience after the healing. She shut her eyes, and with Rose's hands on her head she was able to relax very quickly. She heard Rose discuss the rigidity of her spine with Max."'[23] She then described how Rose discussed a dark area below her ribs on the left side to Cade. Norah revealed later that she had been born with polycystic kidney disease, a fact of which Gladden was unaware. What was extraordinary for the audience to observe was they could not only see, by the coloured flashing lights, the healing energy transferred to the healee; they could also observe Rose Gladden's inner states being transformed - from meditation, relaxation and then steadily falling into the altered state of consciousness. Within a few minutes, Gladden was producing strong alpha waves, and gradually Norah relaxed into these alpha waves too. It seemed that the healer could transform the healee's state, in addition to her own.

In our project with the creative group, we have also experimented with technology and healing, by scanning people's auras. The results of our aura photography are in the colour section of this book. With 2 members of the group, healers present also tried giving healing while both healer and healee were attached to sensors, and then photographed the changes to the auras as a result. The difference in colour seemed to produce orange with Reiki healing and a deeper blue with spiritual healing. This colour ties in with Sir Arthur Conan Doyle's assertion that spiritual healing energy is blue - see page 60. More discussion about this part of our project can be seen in Chapter 4.

Rose Gladden continued to work with her husband at her own healing centre in Letchworth, in her home and they also used an energising technique for objects. She maintained that she could not help everybody, believing that the healee had to work with her and be willing to change. Cade also worked with healers Addie Raeburn, Edgar Chase and Bruce MacManaway in this period.

Harry Edwards (1893 -1976)

The work of Harry Edwards is widely known in the UK, and his ability to fill the Royal Albert Hall with people keen to feel his healing energy was proof of public recognition of his work. For Edwards, the source of an undoubted power for healing comes from 'a close co-operation with more developed spiritual intelligences in the unseen world.'[24] He

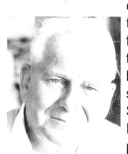

Harry Edwards
Picture courtesy of the Tustees of the Harry Edwards Healing Sanctuary

wrote several books about his work, maintaining that we do survive physical death and influence from beyond the grave can reach us. Edwards discovered a talent for healing in the Middle East during the war, when the local people called him *hakim*, meaning 'healer' because when he cleaned their wounds, they often seemed to heal quicker. His first contact with Spiritualism was at a church in Clements Road, Ilford. He was by no means an easy convert, but his psychic and healing powers soon began to develop more fully. In 1935 he was meditating for a friend who had tuberculosis and he became aware, in his mind's eye, that he had travelled to the hospital. He felt a strange energy go through him. The next day, the friend was making a spontaneous recovery. By 1946 he had bought a house at Shere in order to set up a healing centre. Within two years he was receiving around 3,500 letters a week and, as the number rose to over 9,000, he had to take on extra staff. His public demonstrations grew to fill the Royal Albert Hall with 5,000 people and healers.

Edwards was instrumental in the formation of the National Federation of Spiritual Healers (NFSH) which now has over 7,000 members. The NFSH has long been developing and establishing a relationship with orthodox medicine and has been very successful. There is now a national doctor/healer referral network and many doctors have healers in their surgeries.

When asked to define how he became aware of medical information, Edwards stated that he was the attuned receiver of information; he named 2 guides - the French chemist Louis Pasteur and English surgeon Lord Joseph Lister. Although he credited his healing successes to spirit guides, he did not claim to become any physician, unlike for example George Chapman.

In 1954 a member of the Archbishops' Commission on Divine Healing asked Harry Edwards to put in writing what he believed to be the power and procedure that lay behind spiritual healing.

His beliefs were stated as follows:

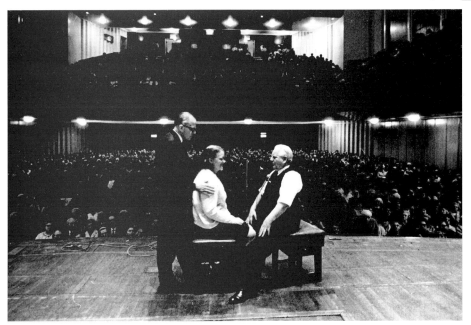

- that spiritual healing comes from God.
- that healers carry out the commandment of Jesus to heal the sick.
- that healers themselves do not posses any healing powers. They are simply the human instruments of God.
- that spiritual healing occurs only within the frame work of God's total laws created for human good.
- that angels may be appointed by God to assist human ministers in the process of spiritual healing.
- Healings do not occur as a result of God's personal intervention on behalf of a particular individual, overriding his established physical laws.
- Divine healing provides demonstrable proof of the human soul and the continuity of life.

Harry Edwards at a packed healing demonstration in the Royal Festival Hall in London. Photo courtesy of the Trustees of the Harry Edwards Healing Sanctuary.

Edwards was a great believer in distant healing, and this is still carried out today in his healing sanctuary in Burrows Lea. He never doubted that man survives physical death and postulates that healing from what he calls 'the spirit realm' is accomplished through a spirit body (the 'etheric' body[*25]), which is closely connected to the physical body. Harry Edwards selected Ray Brown from the audience to

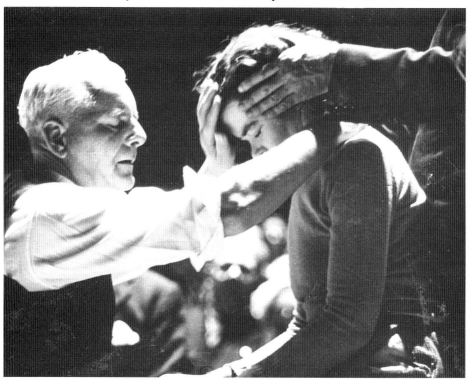

Harry Edwards giving healing to a lady with spondulosis. *Photo courtesy of the Trustees of Harry Edwards Healing Sanctuary*

assist him, at a healing demonstration in Portsmouth when Ray was only 17. Like many healees that Edwards treated in his lifetime, the effect on Ray Brown was similar. The experience simply changed his life.

Ray Brown and Paul

It was 9am on a sunny Wednesday, the 17th of August 2009 and I had made an appointment to visit Ray Brown. Ray Brown is well known, in Britain and abroad, for his work as a spiritual healer who goes into trance, becoming Saint Paul of Tarsus. Ray Brown was voted the UK's Best Known Healer 2007. He is a unique trance medium, who for the past 40 years, has worked with spiritual surgeon Paul, who lived on the earth plane over 2,000 years ago. Together, Paul and Ray have treated thousands of patients with all manner of illnesses from trapped nerves, MS, ME, arthritis, hiatus hernia, back problems and many other conditions. The partnership between Ray and Paul has grown, and gradually they have perfected their technique, so that Ray can be completely removed from his physical body, allowing Paul to remain in our atmosphere for many hours so that he can treat his patients. For over 4 decades, they have successfully treated 1000s of people including doctors, surgeons and celebrities, with a variety of illnesses and medical conditions. Paul specialises in neuro-surgery, but is also a heart surgeon.

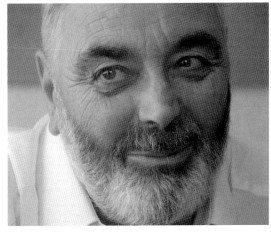

Ray Brown in August 2009 in Hainault
Photo by David Wise

Having worked in the Wednesday group healing clinic at the College of Psychic Studies for many years, I had booked an appointment to meet the man who devised the method we use. At our meditation every week before we begin the healing, we invoke the help of Paul and all the spirit doctors. Finally I was to meet Ray and the doctor he says is working though his body, Saint Paul. I had booked my appointment to interview him, to observe the clinic and also to take photographs. So here I was, accompanied by Maria Spellar, another healer from the Wednesday clinic and David Wise, a photographer who specialises in travel and pinhole photography. When we arrived, I was a bit unsure as to whether I would be meeting Ray and/or Paul.

We met Ray and his wife, Gillian. Ray and Gillian ooze warmth and welcome. "Cup of tea?" Gillian asked us on our arrival. When he had settled down, all my formulated questions to ask Ray about this life disappeared. We just spoke about what had led him to becoming Ray Brown, spiritual healer through whom Paul (of Tarsus) works, while Ray is in trance. Most of us know from the Bible that St Paul underwent a conversion on the road to Damascus, quoted here from Paul himself, at the time. Prior to his conversion to Christianity, Paul was a Pharisee who "violently persecuted" the followers of Jesus.

"You have heard, no doubt, of my earlier life in Judaism. I was violently persecuting the church of God and was trying to destroy it. I advanced in Judaism beyond many among my people of the same age, for I was far more zealous for the traditions of my ancestors."
(Paul's Letter to the Galatians 1:13-14).

Paul's conversion on the road to Damascus occurred after Jesus's crucifixion, and the accounts of Paul's conversion experience describe it as miraculous, supernatural, or otherwise revelatory in nature. A light from heaven flashed around him.

"He fell to the ground and heard a voice say to him, "Saul, Saul, why do you persecute me?' 'Who are you, Lord?' Saul asked. 'I am Jesus, whom you are persecuting," he replied. "Now get up and go into the city, and you will be told what you must do." The men travelling with Saul stood there speechless; they heard the sound but did not see anyone. Saul got up from the ground, but when he opened his eyes he could see nothing. So they led him by the hand into Damascus.

For three days he was blind, and did not eat or drink anything. In Damascus there was a disciple named Ananias. The Lord called to him in a vision, 'Ananias!' 'Yes, Lord," he answered. The Lord told him, 'Go to the house of Judas and ask for a man from Tarsus named Saul, for he is praying. In a vision he has seen a man named Ananias come and place his hands on him to restore his sight.' 'Lord' Ananias answered, 'I have heard many reports about this man and all the harm he has done to your saints in Jerusalem. And he has come here with authority from the chief priests to arrest all who call on your name.' But the Lord said to Ananias, 'Go! This man is my chosen

instrument to carry my name before the Gentiles and their kings and before the people of Israel. I will show him how much he must suffer for my name.'
Then Ananias went to the house and entered it. Placing his hands on Saul, he said, 'Brother Saul, the Lord—Jesus, who appeared to you on the road as you were coming here—has sent me so that you may see again and be filled with the Holy Spirit.' Immediately, something like scales fell from Saul's eyes, and he could see again. He got up and was baptized, and after taking some food, he regained his strength."
(Acts of the Apostles 9:3-19).

I had re-read the piece prior to this visit and I was very curious to interview somebody with a 2,000 year old viewpoint and who has undergone such a major shift in consciousness. Unsure how to start, Ray suggested that we could speak to him first, then after Ray had gone into trance, we could watch Paul at work in the clinic. Ray has an unassuming air about him that I really liked and a good sense of humour. Quite modest and self-effacing, I felt quite comfortable in his presence, although I found that I was very nervous too. I was afraid of wasting his time, of asking the wrong question and so on. I realised this was my own ego interfering and that actually if I relaxed, the right questions would come; so I did.

Pinhole photograph of healers Ray Brown and his wife Gillian in August 2009 at their Hainault clinic. *Photo by David Wise.*

Ray Brown has been involved in healing for many years. When he first started, healing was illegal in many parts of Europe. It still is to this day in France and in Germany, where practitioners need medical qualifications to practise. Ray points out that in the Channel Islands, laws still existed against 'witchcraft' until fairly recently. When he was a teenager, Ray became a member of the Christopher West Healing Group. Ray explained that he was the youngest member of the group. George Jones, the leader of the group, gave him a message that a spirit doctor would join him. Jones' guide, Dr Hoist, explained to Ray that he should train in trance. In the 1960s this was very unusual. Healing was normally done by the laying on of hands. 'We were allowing the power of healing to pass through our bodies without them being taken over'[*26] Ray says in "A Mere Grain of Sand", his biography.

When I questioned Ray about the difference with this type of healing and working with Paul, he was emphatic that Paul is quite different – he is a spiritual doctor who carries out surgical operations through Ray, while Ray is in trance. For people unfamiliar with trance, it is defined as "a half-conscious state characterised by an absence of response to external stimuli, typically as induced by hypnosis or entered by a medium". (Oxford Dictionary.) Even for somebody with years of experience as a healer who works in a clinic devised by Paul, I wondered how this would look and was increasingly keen to see Paul at work.

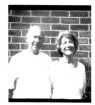

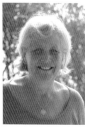

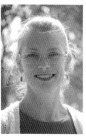

While watching a demonstration in Portsmouth by the renowned healer, Harry Edwards, Ray was chosen from the audience to assist him while healing a client. Ray described this experience to us. "Harry Edwards asked me to come up and help him onstage. I was the youngest member of the Christopher West healing group so this was a great honour for me. The woman was in a wheel-chair. Harry asked me to put my hands on her knees, while he worked on her spine." Then Edwards asked him to let go and told the woman "You can walk now." She denied it and Edwards helped her to stand up. Ray said "She walked! It sold me on healing." For Ray, this was a crucial moment when he decided that his own healing powers needed to find a new method. The Christopher West healing group was not exactly what he needed. So he experimented.

Ray Brown and Paul's individual healing method is very different from the method devised by Paul for group contact healing. I asked Ray why he had set up group healing clinics such as the Wednesday clinic in the College of Psychic Studies. 'It was Paul's idea to spread

Helpers and Healers at Ray Brown's clinics from the top:
1. Alan and Pat Macdonald at Hainault clinic
2. Carol Little and
3. Debbie Thomas at Brighton clinic
Photos by David Wise

this healing all over the world' explained Ray. 'Our work is very different. The clinics are separate from us, but inspired by this method.' The group method was devised by Paul, to ensure that people can access healing frequently, which will help them to improve in the intervals between healing at Ray's clinics and their next appointment. Ray and Paul were aware that people often can't travel to the clinics with ease and Paul wanted this type of healing to be widely available. Often Ray will advise people to attend another clinic. 'Ray and Paul are the doctors and the clinic healers are the nurses' explained Gillian, Ray's wife. Gillian works as a healer in her own right and sometimes assists Paul when required.

Ray Brown, like many healers in this book and in the history of healing, has experienced illness from an early age. He was born on the 4th of May 1946, the second child of Ivor and Marcia Brown. His childhood was spent on an old RAF base near Stratford-upon-Avon. Shortly after starting school, Ray contracted tuberculosis. As it is very infectious, Ray was removed from school and put in a hospital in Stratford-upon-Avon. While talking to us, he lamented his lack of formal education, as a result of being removed from school because of his illness. He also described running away from the nurse who visited him weekly to give him injections and his attempts to hide under the bed or wherever he could! By the time Ray was 7, his mother had left his violent father and met a new partner Bob, and the family moved to Portsmouth, for the benefit of Ray's health. Ray remembers frequent out-of-body experiences in his childhood, aged between 5 and 10. Marcia, Ray's mum was frequently on edge when Ray used to describe what she had put in Bob's sandwiches, as he had been in bed at the time when she was making them. Ray describes with a giggle how surprised she was, as he wandered round the house on his nocturnal travels. Ray believes that these out-of-body experiences were a preparation for his work to come.

Ray comments that it has not been easy. "Paul got me into a lot of problems with my first wife." This was because

Paul frequently felt compelled to get Ray to research, in libraries, on a search for knowledge instead of getting the shopping, for example. Ray can remember getting home to his first wife on one occasion and getting an earful for the delay. By the time the library shut and Ray came to, he couldn't really account for the time and realised that he had no shopping and he was in big trouble. Ray describes his experience of working with Paul as "I'm just the oily rag." Paul is the doctor and the expert and Ray describes how he didn't realise what he was "putting my neck into." He found it hard to accept the idea of Paul.

By this time, Gillian Brown was looking at her watch. It was obvious that Ray was warming up to us and was showing us pictures of his childhood in his book but that Gillian was aware that clients would soon be arriving. 'It's almost time' she reminded him. At this stage, Ray sat himself in a corner of the room and began to close his eyes and attune. Paul was about to arrive. Watching Ray transform to Paul was a bit odd too. One minute Ray is chatting away happily; the next, Gillian is looking at her watch and saying 'It's time now.' She has worked with Ray and Paul for many years now and also has her own healing guides. Gillian says she has to keep track of the timing. 'Ray needs to eat and to take a trip to the loo now and then and to have a cup of tea, like most normal people' she comments. Paul is aware of these physical needs, and slightly protected by being inside Ray's body. The spirit doctors do not have this luxury and remain very vulnerable to the 'treacle' atmosphere of this planet, as described by Paul. I can feel his need to start his healing work. It's not that we are unwelcome but he needs to get started. I begin to understand the strain this must put on Ray's physical body. Imagine if you permitted another soul to enter into your human body and to do it for 7 hours at a time. You agree to it because with this soul, you can send physical relief to many, many people. It's the physical dimension of it that intrigues me. By this time, Gillian Brown was aware that clients would soon be arriving. I need to know a bit more about the healing method so I ask Paul.

Paul

There is actually something very different about the man sitting before me now. It's hard to describe but he sounds different when speaking; his speech is slower, more thoughtful. Later I scan each and every photograph to see if I can confirm my feeling that his eye colour has changed! Gillian Brown really notices the difference. Paul confesses that 'This is my first time on the Earth plane as a spirit. We were both young, I was young.' Paul was discussing reincarnation and the way that he had decided to come back as Paul, the spirit doctor. Ray and Paul's biography 'A mere grain of sand' details life after death and its many levels. Paul explained that the Council had asked him if he would continue this healing work, down on Earth. Paul asked if he could choose his time, place and person. He wanted somebody like Raymond, who he described as having a 'simple family background.'

Paul says that the 'quickening' of 3 months is when spirit comes into the body. Questioned in his book "A Mere Grain of Sand" he states that the life force joins the foetus at 3 months and that God is the life force of this Earth. Paul sees no reason for reincarnation. In fact, he stressed that he believes we should not come back. "This is the only life, if we choose not to reincarnate' reiterated Paul. According to him, there are completely new souls waiting to come but of course, this is impossible as we all are all queuing up to return. Paul has described different levels after death in great detail in his biography. Level 1, the first stage after dying, is whatever you want it to be, but as you progress in spirit, you shed your Earthly ties.'[27] He also stresses that reincarnation does occur but that this is not his teaching. The advice made sense to me.

We need to live our lives now as our only ones. There is no second chance. We should let new beings arrive to help us to change what needs to be done. There is a need for new blood, so to speak. This is when I felt Paul with utmost certainty speaking as if we are almost arrogant to want to come back again and again. I agree, particularly when I observe how little we have learned as a race. Paul described life 2,000 years ago and said the human race then had famine, greed, murder and war. 'And what has changed?' he queried looking at me most intensely, straight at me with unflinching eyes.

'To be honest, very little' was all I could respond. I look at the news headlines for 2009 and 2010, scan through them in their horrifying bold text. Bankers ruin the country, with their greed and speculation. The economy stumbles through mistakes and society seems to relish only finance and materialism. Then the MPs hit the headlines, with their expenses scandal. Politicians pay for their moat to be cleared, for their second homes, for their gardens to be planted with exotic flowers, all paid for by the tax payer. Israel is bombing Palestinians and vice versa, and are both declared guilty of offences by the United Nations. Global warming is seen as a huge threat an awful lot of people, who clamour for action, yet few politicians were prepared to put themselves in the unpopular position of having to cut carbon emissions at the Copenhagen Summit. People continue to fly and to drive, knowing we are damaging our atmosphere. Little boys are shot dead and tortured by other little boys and even more shockingly, by their carers A mother commits suicide with her daughter, after being bullied by teenagers for years. Added to this we have bloody war in Afghanistan, and Pakistan is in turmoil. Not to mind an inquiry into a possibly illegal war in Iraq with interviews and public appearance by our then Prime Minister, who led us in the 'war against terror' using violence and no regrets, even for lost human life. How little human nature changes, even with a 2,000 year old perspective.

Of course, I have my own particular issue and it concerns the natural world, Mother Earth, nature, the trees and the skies from which we breathe. I questioned Paul about healing for our planet Earth. In his book, he asks "What are we doing to our mother Earth?" As I wax lyrical about how we can send the same universal love energy to trees and to the earth, as we do to people, he smiles. Paul advises me to find my pathway, says he

Ray Brown's Hainault and Brighton Clinics
The pictures on pages 91-92 show the sequence of various healing sessions with Ray Brown and Paul.

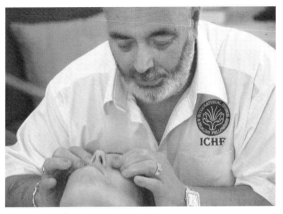

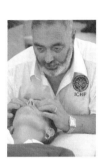

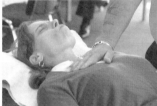

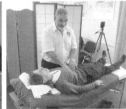

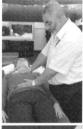

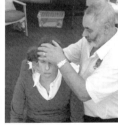

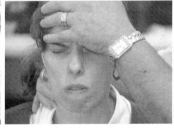

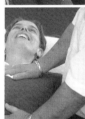

From top, left to right: Ray Brown working with Maria Spellar in his Brighton clinic in September 2009.
Photos by David Wise

would be wrong to judge anybody. That I should do what I feel is right and it must be my own pathway. This leads to natural gap for breath. Ray and Paul are keen to start work. Above and on the next page, you can see Ray and Paul working with various visitors to their clinics in Hainault and Brighton. A description of Paul's group healing method follows on page 93.
Testimonials can be found at the end of Chapter 3.

Left to right:
Ray Brown
working with
Kelly Patrick
and healer
Carol Little at
his Brighton
clinic, 2009.

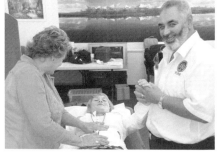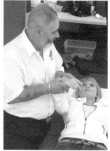

Left to right:
Kelly Patrick
at a healing
session with
Ray Brown
and Paul in
Brighton, 2009.
*Photos by
David Wise*

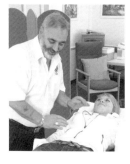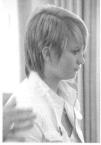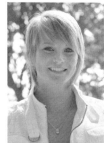

Left to right:
Anna Wells
with Ray Brown
and Paul in
Hainault,
August 2009.
*Photos by
David Wise*

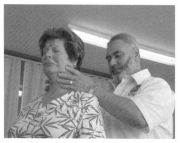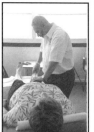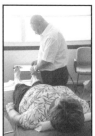

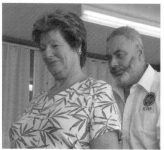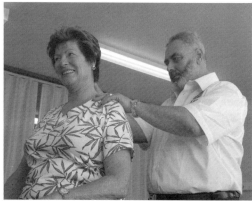

Paul's group healing method

The healing which I devised requires 3 healers. There are 3 separate healing rays into the body. This method means that there is no ego between the 3 healers. The healing energy comes as one, and everybody must be in harmony. The healing rays come through spirit doctors. As soon as they make contact with the healer in the group, the energy passes from them to the healer and then into the healee's body.

The strength of the ray can be altered, depending on the ailment treated. It is also necessary to ask spirit to come in advance. Paul explains that Spirits do not come down from on high. We pass from our own dimension, which is Spirit, into your dimension, the Earth plane. For this reason, healers need to give notice of their intention to heal and to prepare themselves. At the College of Psychic Studies, June Frost the Clinic Leader asks everybody to prepare the night before and to alert spirit to make any connections necessary. Paul continues 'We change spirit doctors every 2 clients. The spirits are vulnerable to earthly atmospheres.'

Paul suggests colours for people when they first come to see him. These are recorded by Gillian on a file about the person and afterwards, if people go to a group healing clinic, they can inform the healers of the colours chosen for them by Paul. The colours represent a strength of the ray. Working from violet/purple as the strongest, red/orange as less strong and so on downwards to blue, green and yellow as the weakest, Paul assigns colours to each healer on the couch, starting with healer 1 on the head, healer 2 on the upper chest and abdomen and Healer 3, one of whose hands is between Healer 2 and the lowest hand is on the abdomen. Please see photograph on page 101.

Paul stressed that all healers should send pastel colours, not strong, vivid ones, as colour strength can be intensified by the spirits but not changed. Paul explains that if a healer sends too strong a colour, then the spirit doctors cannot change this. Paul stressed that if a healee has not been to see him to get colours, then healers in clinics should hold a pastel colour strong in their minds when sending healing during this method. He clarifies that this is not colour healing. The healing session lasts for only 4 minutes. In the College of Psychic Studies, this is timed to 4 minutes for each healee.

4 healers can be used to help cancer patients .

This brief history of healing cannot hope to list and interview all the names and personalities involved in healing throughout history. Some deserve mention even by name only, such as Jose Pogson, Edgar Chase, Major Bruce MacManaway, Swami Prakashanand, and Addie Raeburn, all of whom worked with Max Cade. Other names include the Worralls, Oskar Estebany and Matthew Manning. I have read much about the work of John Mc-Cain in the north of England. My own healer, Angela Palmer, works and teaches in the College, and for many years has also been the person I go to for healing, for which I am truly grateful. Sue Allen was interviewed for this book on the subject of auras and her healing and psychic work has been well documented on radio and in her own book. I recently attended workshops by Angie Buxton-King and Graham King, who have made such great efforts to get healing accepted into NHS hospitals. Their pioneering work in University College London Hospital is simply an inspiration. Dr Dolores Kreiger's 'Therapeutic Touch' has been a thought provoking work for so many nurses in the US and all over the world. Dr Daniel J Benor's books have widened my knowlege of healing all over the globe. The author has attempted to contact many healers and their families. I've carefully selected those with any connection to the College of Psychic Studies, when in doubt. Any omissions are mine. If you would like any healers to be included in any future reprints, the author would be very grateful if you could get in touch with details.

NOTES

*1 – Marilyn Ferguson, The Aquarian Conspiracy.

*2 – The Maya used a shamanic liquer called balché to induce trances. It is derived from a honey from xtabentún – a vining morning glory (Latin: Turbina corymbosa). It has been shown to be rich in psychotropic ergoline alkaloids. This mead, combined with the bark of the balché tree (Lonchocarpus violaceus, which is added during fermentation was then used in ceremonies. The drunkenness reported by the Spanish was undoubtedly related to an aspect of Maya ritual not well described in the ethnohistorical documents: divination, or ritual acts designed to communicate directly with supernatural powers. Divination is used to foretell future events and to determine causes for events otherwise not understood, the reasons for illness, misfortune, and so forth…. But the ancient Maya also seem to have used substances that altered the individual's normal state of consciousness, almost certainly as a part of divinatory ritual. Thus the ingestion of narcotics, hallucinogens and other psychometric substances was seen as a way to transform existence and to meet or communicate with unseen powers….The Maya, like most Mesoamerican peoples, made fermented alcoholic beverages, using maize and agave (pulque); especially favoured for ritual purposes was the drink balche, made from fermented honey and the bark of the balche tree (Lonchocarpus longistylis).The Ancient Maya, Sylvanus G Morley, George W Brainerd, 4th edition. Original published 1946 by SG Morely.

*3 World Tree. A universal symbol. See 'The Tree of Life' by Roger Cook.

*4 Only 3 (possibly 4) manuscripts have survived the burning of native literature and art as a result of the Spanish conquest. Named after the cities where they are now in musuems, the surviving manuscripts are known as the Paris Codex, The Dresden Codex and the Madrid Codex. Michael D Coe believes that the Grolier Codex is also a genuine Codex of the Maya.

*5 For some members of this group, spirituality is embodied in their church, like Gill, Derrick and James who run a group for people with Cerebellar Ataxia

*6 'The Blue Island' page xii, introduction by Arthur Conan Doyle

*7 WT Stead frontispiece, with Stead's face beside his daughter's

*8 p73 'The Blue Island' by W T Stead

*9 Powers of Healing, p11

*10 Maxwell Cade's research work in biofeedback, states of consciousness etc is discussed in more detail in Chapter 4.

*11 Ayahuasca was explored as a treatment for a medical diagnosis by Donald M. Topping, Ph.D.Professor Emeritus, University of Hawaii, who was President of the Drug Policy Forum of Hawaii.

*12 Jeremy Narby, 'The Cosmic Serpent' quotes research by Luna (1984, p179-180) in which spirits present themselves during dreams and visions; they show how to diagnose illness, what plants to use and how, the proper use of tobacco smoke, how to suck out the illness or restore the spirit to a patient.

*13 In 'Spiritual Healing' Dr Daniel J Benor comments that "the mechanical and biochemical models" favoured by conventional medicine cannot explain many aspects of health and illness. The mind and body are intimately linked, each influencing the other eg hypnotic and post anaesthetic suggestion can dramatically alleviate pain and other post-surgical discoforts and complications". (Daniel J Benor P6)

*14 Dr Bernie Siegel, who works with groups of cancer patients in his ECaP programme for Exceptional Cancer Patients. He is also the author of best-seller 'Love, Medicine and Miracles'.

*15 David Furlong, The Complete Healer, 1995. p190-91.

*16 The I Ching: The Book of Change is an ancient divinatory tradition from China. See the Richard Wilhelm Translation in Index 1.

*17 Citation from Wikipedia (http://en.wikipedia.org/wiki/Asclepius)

*18 Greatrakes is discussed in detail in 'The seven levels of healing' by Lilla Bek and Philppa Pullar, see Index 1.

*19 Ray and Gillian Brown, A mere grain of sand. p168, see Index 1.

*20 Edward Cayce, Powers of Healing, p31.

*21 A Graham Ikin, Studies in Spiritual Healing.

*22 Wrekin Trust Annual Conference at Loughborough in 1977. Described in 'The Awakened Mind' Cade & Coxhead, see Index 1.

*23 David Harvey, The Power to Heal, p93-4.

*24 A Graham Ikin, Studies in Spiritual Healing p40.

*25 The 'etheric body' is a layer of the aura. Healers often work on this layer. It can be seen in thermal imaging, Kirlian photography and aura photography. Please see chapter 4 for more details about the aura.

*26 A mere grain of sand, Ray and Gillian Brown. p18

*27 A mere grain of sand, Ray and Gillian Brown. p165

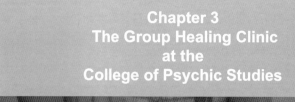

Chapter 3
The Group Healing Clinic
at the
College of Psychic Studies

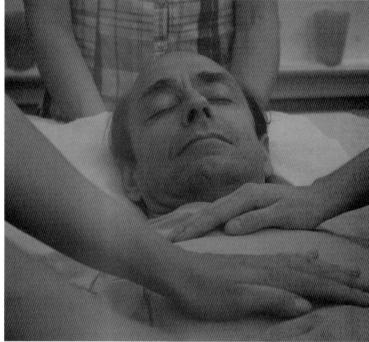

Jonathon, a member of the group during a healing session at the Group Healing Clinic in 2009. *Photo by Derek Wilkinson*

The deeper the healer's understanding of self, the deeper the resonance with the healee's problems
˙Dolores Krieger,[1] *Therapeutic Touch*

The patient must ultimately be responsible for his own system, so he must be helped to help himself - so that he will not be dependent on his healer. Lilla Bek and Philippa Pullar,[2]
The Seven Levels of Healing

95

themomentisnow

Harry Edwards, the famous British spiritual healer wrote in 'The Power of Spiritual Healing'[3] that the purpose of spiritual healing is not only the healing of the sick but also to prevent disease and to awaken man's spiritual consciousness by demonstrating the power of the spirit in this materialistic and scientific age; and our kinship with it. Spiritual Healing, according to the Harry Edwards Healing Sanctuary, is a simple, safe and supportive energy therapy that aims to bring balance to mind/body and soul, as well as to stimulate the body's own natural healing ability. The healer links to the healing energy in a method called 'attunement' and is a channel through which the healing energy flows to the person/animal who may or may not be present. It is complementary to all forms of treatment, as it is non invasive and patients are always encouraged to seek medical advice for their conditions. You do not have to be ill to benefit from Spiritual Healing as it also supports good health and well being.

For those who have experienced healing, this explanation will seem simplistic, as the experience is so vast and on so many levels and very difficult to articulate in words, like trying to capture a dream. To those who have not experienced healing, it is often the same old story that healers hear. "I don't believe in all that stuff" on the one hand and then "I'm here because I've tried everything else" and all shades in between. Often healing is tried in desperation, because nothing else works.

To quote Dr Angela Watkins, who established this clinic, "The absolute last thing I tried was healing. I had tried everything else." Healers accept anybody who wants healing including the doubters, the lost causes, the terminally and chronically ill, sometimes because the medical profession has been unable to help them apart from offering more drugs, putting up with it and even giving up. It should be noted however, that healing is also of benefit to people who are in good health; the benefit from spiritual healing is that it balances energy centres and helps well being.

This chapter looks in detail at the people behind the Group Contact Healing Clinic in the College of Psychic Studies in London, set up by Dr Angela Watkins assisted by June Frost, Clinic Leader. The stories of the people involved show that often the healer must go through their own healing journey. To quote one of the healers, Beulah Hudson, "There's no Ivory Tower for us!"

June Frost describes how healing works. ""We work with unconditional love, which comes from the highest and purest good. This healing energy of love flows through the body, cleansing and clearing away any negative energies such as sadness, depression, anger, guilt, etc. After a few sessions of healing we begin to feel stronger and more able, mentally and spiritually to take charge of ourselves and make our own decisions without depending on others. Many clients who have received healing say that their pain has receded or disappeared completely."

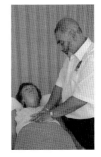

Ray Brown, spiritual healer, works in trance with his spirit doctor Paul, seen here working in his Hainault clinic in Essex in 2009.

Dolores Krieger the nurse who developed Therapeutic Touch[1], describes how healers feel when they touch the *auras* (ie the electromagnetic field which surround the body) of clients. The major sensations that healers have said they feel are similar to what clients say they feel - heat, cold, tingling, pressure, electric shocks or pulsations. She describes how one of these sensations, that of the feeling of pressure seems to be indicative of "a kind of static condition in the field; perhaps the best description might be the word 'congestion' as that word is used in the literature on acupuncture to indicate a blockage in the meridians through which the *chi*, or vital energy, flows through the body."

A biophysicist who took one of Dolores' workshops told her that the reason for this feeling was that, as the hands move over the affected areas of the field, they pick up positive ions. Positive ions are formed when an atom loses an electron for some reason. Although the effects of ionisation on human physiology have been studied for over 90 years, the understanding is still in its infancy. Positive ion loading has been noted in crowded and congested locations where the feelings of lethargy, headache, irritability and symptoms of stemming from inflammation of the mucosal tissues have been noted to prevail. On the other hand, a prevalence of negative ions has been noted in areas in which people report feelings of well being, such as sites near waterfalls and in mountainous terrain.

Paul, Ray Brown's spirit doctor, devised this group contact healing method over a period of 30 years, which consists of three healers working together to give healing to the client who is lying on a couch. Please see photo opposite for more information about positioning of hands etc. The client lies on the couch on their back and then three healers place their hands on or near the central nervous system. Healer 1 places both hands behind the head, fingers touching the back of the neck on either side of the brain stem and healers 2 and 3 place their hands across the upper chest and the abdomen, over sections of the spinal cord. This healing only needs to be given for 4 minutes, as it is so powerful.

Paul chose and taught 16 healers how to administer this contact healing method. One of these was Dr Angela Watkins PhD, SRN, ONC (a College of Psychic Studies healer, tutor and medium), who then taught the method at workshops at the College. Susanna McInerney, the then President, agreed to her opening a contact healing clinic at the college after receiving this healing herself, as well as the healing tutors. Other clinics were opened by Angela in Wandsworth, Barnes and East Sheen. The Group Contact Healing Clinic led by Dr Angela Watkins and June Frost, received the first clients on 17 March 2003, giving healing to eight clients. The clinic proved to be very popular and by September 2004 the clinic was giving healing to approximately 30 clients at each session. Many requests have been made by clients since then, for the clinic to extend through the afternoon and operate for the same hours as the Monday clinic. Max Eames, the president, has given permission in principle for this extension and it is now a matter of organisation.

The clinic operates in a very safe, supportive way, helped by the strength and wisdom of the Clinic Leader,

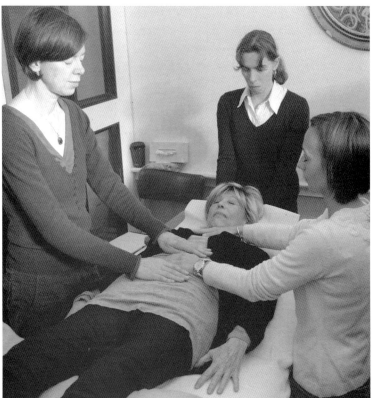

Group Healing Method

Healer 1 (at the head) Maria Spellar, places hands at the base of the brain stem, behind the neck. Healer 2 (right) Valerie Renaud, places hands as shown, one on the upper chest and the other on the abdomen. Healer 3 (left) Beulah Hudson, places her hands on either side of healer 2. The healing session is timed to exactly 4 minutes, as prescribed by Ray Brown. *Photo David Wise*

June Frost. When interviewing Ray Brown and Paul about this method, he could not stress enough just how important it is for the clinic leader to be without ego and very strong. Lucy, one of the healers commented that this clinic has a very special quality; for her, this is embodied in the kindness and firmness of the clinic leader but also the fact that she thinks of the little things. "No other clinic I work in has biscuits!" Lucy commented with a smile and this small point is actually very important to those who work in the clinic. Some healers have worked alongside June for years and new healers join the clinic all the time; some for a trial and others who find this method is the best one for them and who stay longer.

Many of us like the aspect of working with other healers in a group rather than working individually with clients, feeling the companionship and also the strength of working with like-minded souls. The room itself seems to take on a shiny, buzzing feeling once the clinic has been going for an hour and this is tangible both to clients coming in to reception and to the healers working in the clinic. Dr Angela Watkins describes this group healing method as "holistic, subtle and a deep experience on every level – emotional, physical and spiritual.'

The positive results of using this method of healing are numerous. Feedback forms from clients have shown that many clients preferred this method – see some of their comments at the end of this chapter. Clients feel very supported by three healers using three rays of energy and the effect was long lasting. The contact healing clinic has always encouraged probationer healers from the College of Psychic Studies accreditation healing course to use their gift alongside trained healers in this supervised and professionally run clinic. This method of healing has been included in the College of Psychic Studies healing syllabus since 2007.

There are many stories of how this clinic came to be. Below are the stories of the healers who have worked in the clinic.

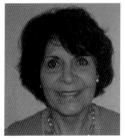

Angela Watkins

Until I was 45, I was healthy, with endless energy. I had a lovely husband and two children and I played tennis and hockey and people always commented on my energy levels, how energetic I was. Then I had a virus in a heart muscle and I had two near death experiences. This led to chronic fatigue syndrome, ME. I was exhausted, I lost weight, I had multiple food allergies and Irritable Bowel Syndrome. I was too exhausted by the illness to go back to my work (as a nurse). I'd go to conferences with doctors and specialists and leave them feeling worse than when I went in. I had been to all the best doctors in Harley Street and Wimpole Street. The worst thing was that I never met anybody who got over it, but I decided I was not going to accept that I was going to stay like it! I had tried everything, including acupuncture. This was the best of all the treatments and I felt a bit better but the absolute last thing I tried was healing. I had tried everything else.

After my heart arrythmia, I had a relapse. I felt so ill that I felt as if my brain was cooking. I was driving one day, on my way to Richmond. I saw a sign on a placard and it said 'Spiritual Healing'. I had no idea what it was, I'd never tried it, I knew nothing about it at all. So I went in. This was Richmond Healing Clinic. When I got there the healers were meditating and somebody told me to sit down, that one of them would come over for me when they were ready. A lovely German lady came over to me. I knew she would, before she came. I could see light around her head. I was a nurse but I had no idea what would happen. They didn't teach things like healing then in nursing. I returned to the clinic several times and eventually, I told this German lady about what was psychically happening, because my spirit grandmother kept coming. "I wondered when you would tell me! They've been waiting for you."

I felt so good after the healing that eventually I decided that I had to learn how to do it myself, as a way of saying thank you. The illness was all for a reason. My heart actually stopped several times. I knew it but I was in all this light, higher than my body; an out-of-body experience. My heart was beating wildly - 156 beats per minute. The doctors had previously told me "Don't call a doctor. Call an ambulance so that they can work on you in the ambulance." So I did. This voice told me to "Get them to help you on the way." I suppose I knew that I wouldn't survive unless I called the ambulance. I wasn't scared. I knew I had to come back for my children. I suppose it was all connected to the death of my husband (2 years before). At the time, I couldn't understand it. "Where's he gone?" I asked my local vicar. I was sad, don't get me wrong, but I asked him why he thought it had happened to my family and me. He was very wise. "Maybe this has happened as an example to other people."

I'd been to see Ray Brown[4] myself several times for

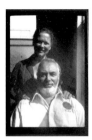

Ray and Gillian Brown at their Hainault Clinic in August 2009

myself and I'd taken lots and lots of people to visit him. I was doing a lot of research into healing. I just had to know all about it. I wanted to understand it. Ray just invited me to go to wherever he was living at the time, to learn how to do the group contact healing work. He told me it had taken him 30 years to devise a method. The (spirit) doctors can come for each individual healing client and stay in the clinic but only for 4 minutes. Only 4 minutes is required to use these subtle and deep 3 rays of energy. They don't need to be there any longer. You can stay there another 10 minutes, but they are no longer there after 4 minutes.

I enjoy a challenge and setting things up. My job in this clinic was to do that, to set it up with the right clinic leader. I've also lost any fear. After my heart problems, my children bought me a mobile and I used to worry about losing the phone and one day I threw it into a bush when I was out walking! On my healing course, lots of students were feeling tingling and heat when giving healing. I felt none of those so I asked my tutor. She replied "You've been doing it all your life. It's not extraordinary to you. You've been living it."

June Frost's story

At a very early age I was able to see the energy field (aura[*3]) around people, and remember being able to see the emotions of both love and fear. I would cuddle into my mother tightly until I was right inside her aura, which was filled with a very strong and protective love. During the (Second World) war, when the air raid sirens warned of an attack, I remember the colour for fear. It was grey, translucent and shot up from the feet to just above the heads of the children who were playing outside. Within about 10 seconds the road would empty, as the children rushed home.

During my childhood I had many illnesses, including diptheria, when I was in hospital for 9 weeks. I had my thirteenth birthday in hospital, suffering from appendicitis, peritonitis, septic tonsillitis, gastric 'flu and a touch of scarlet fever, all at once. The doctors in King's College

Hospital in London told my parents not to hold out any hope, but they did a wonderful job and I had a new lease of healthier life after this. They were so loving and caring that the Sister even made a birthday cake for me at home in her own time! I have always been grateful to the doctors and nurses for saving my life.

When my mother became ill, the GP was unable to offer her any help and simply said 'Look around, what medicine would you like?' because he didn't know how to treat her. I heard about a healer, and suggested to my mother that she went to see one. However, her strict Catholic upbringing led her to believe that healing was the work of the devil and she would have none of it. As the years went by I became interested in

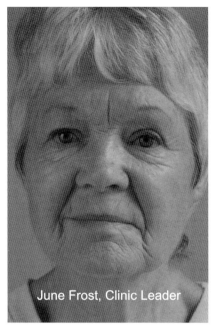

June Frost, Clinic Leader

healing and attempted to send her healing, but she made me promise not to do it again.

After my parents died I went to a medium, who told me that my father said I was meant to be a healer, and gave me the name and address of the College of Psychic Studies. I laughed at the idea and forgot about all about this until about 3 months later, when I went to a different medium, who gave me exactly the same message. That stopped me in my tracks and really made me think. Some time later, I telephoned the College of Psychic Studies and asked to be out on the list for a healing / psychic development course, but they had no vacancies left. A little while later I received a call from them, saying that someone had dropped out and inviting me to come for an interview, before being accepted on the course.

I took the NFSH[*5] healing accreditation course and the College of Psychic Studies healing accreditation course. Healing has changed my life completely and has filled an empty spiritual hole within me. I always knew that there was something else I should be doing, but did not know what it was until I started channelling healing. I worked in the Monday healing clinic (in the college) for four and a half years, three years as clinic leader, during which time the clinic was split into the morning and afternoon clinics and expanded from 2 hours to 5 hours. After this I had a powerful feeling that my work there was finished and I knew that I was meant to do something else but did not know what that would be. Shortly after I had left the clinic Angela Watkins telephoned me and said she was setting up the Group Contact Healing Clinic. She asked me if I would be the leader and I said that I did not want to lead the clinic, which entailed clerical work, arranging rotas etc but would be happy to work as a healer. 3 of us demonstrated the healing on Suzanna McInerney, the then President, who was impressed with the healing and confirmed that this clinic could commence. She assumed that I would be leading the clinic, and somehow I found myself agreeing to this.

Prior to this, I had been suffering with stomach pains for about 2 years, after a bout of *Heliobacter pylori*, although tests proved that medication had killed the germ. I went to see Ray Brown (Paul), who devised the group contact method of healing. After about 5 visits to him, the pain had disappeared and he also released some trapped

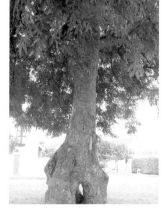

nerves in my ribs! I was walking on air and had forgotten what it was like to be free of pain!

I believe that learning to meditate is very important, since it opens the door to spiritual knowledge and importantly learning what makes us tick ourselves. During one meditation, I saw a big strong tree with a hole in the side and a wooden seat around the tree. I found myself going through the hole, into the tree and being made aware that the tree was both mother and father to all the insects and animals who lived within it, protecting them with love. Then a storm came and lightning shot across the sky. The tree opened its branches and drew

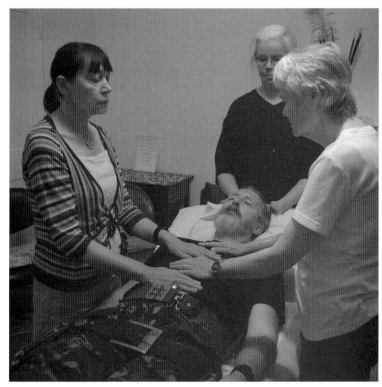

Healing in the Sanctuary with Gordian in July 2009. Healers from the left, Cynthia, at the head Kathy and far right, June Frost, Clinic Leader.

energy and life from this, which invigorated the tree, keeping it strong and healthy. After this, I became the tree and reached out to the heavens with my branches. I felt that I knew everything there was to know and withot any doubt that love and goodness were the most powerful forces in the universe. I came out of the meditation feeling elated, with certain knowlege that there was a vast amount of love and goodness ion the world, infinitely more than one was led to believe, in spite of the negative events which were given top priority in the newspapers and in the news on TV.

I feel that the College of Psychic Studies is the jewel in the crown of spiritual wisdom and is going to be very important on the world stage, as more and more people awaken spiritually and seek more knowledge. The ethos of the college is to train students to their highest potential whether it is healing, psychic development, personal growth etc. As soon as I walk into the college a powerful ambience of goodness and truth permeates the atmosphere and my spirit soars!

The Group Contact Healing Clinic has a very powerful spiritual energy, due to the fact that the healers work in groups of 3. I consider that I am very privileged to work in this happy, friendly, loving atmosphere, where all the members of the clinic are dedicated and work for the highest and purest good.

The Healers' stories follow in alphabetical order. The clinic is run and staffed by volunteers. Healers studying in the College can work alongside accredited healers at the clinic, to gain experience. Accreditation includes a practical, timed demonstration of healing and questions from the panel about the Code of Conduct, to which all healers must adhere. Receptionists sometimes become healers, as in the case of Maria Spellar.

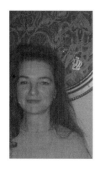

Lucy Aumonier
Whilst on the intensive healing course (at the college), we were introduced to June Frost who talked about the work at the clinic. I was touched by her gentle nature and considerate non judgemental attitude. She showed us how to give the healing specific to this clinic. We worked on June and I was surprised how intense and immediate it was. The next term, a friend who worked there told me how enjoyable it was, so I rang June.

I have experience of dis-ease from my own journey, family and friends. I have been taught to understand what this means on a metaphysical level, which enables me to consider mind, body and spirit, facilitating the client to work from the big picture, rather than the symptom only.

I have worked at several different clinics and this clinic for me works very much for the good of all, which includes the healers, something which is often overlooked. It is professionally run, ensuring we are protected, grounded and working as a group. Each healer has specific interests and backgrounds, bringing further knowledge to our work and because we work in threes this allows debate and continued learning as cases are presented. It is a joyous place of work and healers have often said they love working at this clinic.

There is a real sense of community spirit, which helps not only those who come for healing but everyone involved. Not forgetting the chocolate biscuits! (I mention this because we don't get them in other clinics and it's a reflection of June considering others - which is a hallmark of hers, something nice and personal about her reflects in this clinic, the fact that we have time for tea and chat is a real bonus).

Anya Borta (receptionist)

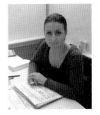

Joining the clinic was like a sign of destiny. I saw the advert by accident on the wall at the college and I was thinking that it would be great to apply, but had some doubts about how I was going to do them both: the clinic and my job. And right at that moment, I received a long awaited call that gave me the news I will be able to do them both. I knew that this was going to be a special experience. The College of Psychic Studies and the Clinic were something I've never done before. I never thought I'd have this kind of opportunity so quickly. It happened all of a sudden. I haven't experienced any illnesses that required special treatment or healing. The healing I receive gave me a balance I didn't have before, made me listen to my body, a thing I haven't felt before and all my friends say that there's a nice energy felt about me. "You are shining!" they say.
Veronica Curry, Aoife Nally and Cherina Tully also work as clinic receptionists.

Ann Brayton Meek

I am a student of healing at the College of Psychic Studies and the opportunity came up for me to join the clinic as a student healer.

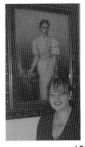

During my life I have had several severe shocks and following the shocks, I've had long periods of depletion lasting as long as seven years at a stretch. It is now thankfully several years ago now. My only debility now is diabetes, which I've had for the last three years.

I am poet in residence at St Ethelburgha's Centre for peace and reconciliaition. I am also a clavical singer, but I don't perform now.

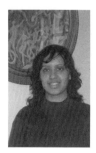

Rosina Chaudry

Whilst studying at the college, we had a session on group healing. I really enjoyed this session and decided that I'd like to volunteer for one of the clinics in the future. It wasn't until I was accredited that I began volunteering at the College. I find working alongside other healers a valuable support network. It's the joint effort that make the sessions so intense and worthwhile.

In my early 20's I became unexpectedly ill with vertigo and fatigue, which lasted for 2 years. Allopathically, the doctors could not find anything physically wrong with me so I began to research and venture into other thought forms and practices to make myself well again.

I began my self-help with affirmations, meditations and visualisations. This proved incredibly helpful and this discovery of self-healing has been a turning point in my life. I fully recovered and went on to do Reiki and the College's accredited healing course. I also became much more active and took up running, hiking and trekking. I have continued on this healing path, using my experience of illness in a positive way by healing others.

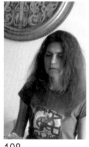

Elena Friedman

I completed the Healing Course at the College of Psychic Studies and I wanted to share my healing abilities with other people who may benefit. I also believed that from practising healing at the clinic, I would further develop my healing abilities. It is a wonderful experience to work with the team of healers when you channel, share and multiply the healing energy and see the patients responding positively. I did not have any experience of being ill. But I have to lead a certain lifestyle of self-discipline to stay healthy. This includes a raw vegan diet, a minimum of 2 litres of water per day and daily yoga practice. And of course, purification of thoughts and intentions. My strongest motivation to work at the healing clinic is an opportunity to share a beautiful loving healing energy. I have seen people change in wonderful ways as a result of our healing and that have been very inspiring and deeply satisfying.

Beulah Hudson
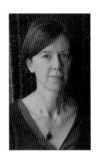
I joined the Wednesday healing clinic during my third module of the accredited healing course, partly to gain experience of healing members of the public, and partly because I liked the sound of the healing method used: working in small groups and visualizing the healing energy in colours. I've been doing this for about a year now and enjoy it very much.

It's great to be able to work in a small group of healers as the energy is intensified. Different healers bring different life experiences and areas of interest in healing and health, so it's good for the clients to have the benefit of our different approaches and advice. Also, the client can choose to see a particular healing group if they wish. The group members are constantly rotated so we are able to work together in different combinations with everyone in the clinic. Because we are working together we have the benefit of learning from each other's different approaches and experience. If one healer in a group has personal experience of the client's situation or health problem, the other healers can learn from the way they help the client.

One of the things I particularly like about the Wednesday healing clinic is that the hands-on healing method is prescribed, so that the healers can focus on channelling the energy. I would say that what brought me to healing was more to do with emotional issues and emotional balance than any physical health problem, lthough I have suffered from an overactive thyroid and hormone imbalances. I have found healing extremely helpful and transformative.

The only thing I would say is that as healers we are forced to deal with our own self-healing issues and this can be difficult at times - there's no ivory tower for us!

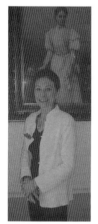

Linda Hinshelwood

I joined the clinic to have an opportunity to practise healing and meet up with like-minded souls. The group healing is special. It has a completely different energy. I can only spare one Wednesday a month because of the day job but I really look forward to that day of the month. It's healing for me too.

I also like being in the college... it has such a wonderful atmosphere and feeling. You can feel it as you walk into the building. I suppose being involved in the clinic means that I still have a link with the college, now that I've passed my accreditation. If I get any inspirational thoughts, I will forward them onto you... I will meditate on it tonight!

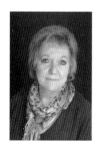

Greta Jenkins

I joined the clinic because after I finished the healing course I wanted to offer my healing to those in need. The Wednesday clinic is excellent - very powerful, collective energies for the clients and for the healers, a good sense of teamwork and collaboration.

My experience of illness is quite extensive. My mother died after an illness when I was 12, my first husband died suddenly after 6 weeks of marriage and my last partner died after a short illness about 15 years ago. I have also been near to many others with differing types of diseases and serious conditions.

However, this has not damaged my capacity to enjoy life and has helped me to really appreciate the time we have on earth! These experiences have obviously made me more aware of life energies, life after death, forces we cannot see, our own place in the universe and how we can use that awareness for good.

Tina Lawlor Mottram

I joined the clinic because I saw an ad on the healers' notice board in the college, asking for healers to join the group healing clinic. I phoned June Frost and agreed that I would come along to try it out. This was in 2004 and I've never looked back. There is something so special about the clinic for me; the meditation for healers before we start, leaving the world outside and making this room full of love and light to enable people to relax and to receive healing and be motivated to heal themselves. We see over 30 people a day; coming and going every 15 minutes. I always feel that the room we work in is protected. Some of the greatest names in mediumship have worked in the college, including Daniel Dunglas Home, whose well-known portrait hangs above the fireplace in the clinic, and this is all part of working in the College.

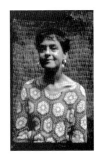

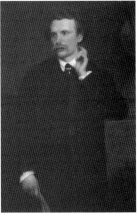

Portrait of
Daniel Home

My first experience of healing was when I was working at a centre in Aranjuez, in Spain, for people with AIDS. People would sit in a circle, holding the hands of the person on either side. I realise now that what I experienced as an electrical shock was actually some healing energy going around the circle. I just couldn't deny that something quite strange had happened and I couldn't explain it. When I came back to the UK, I found the healing clinics in the College and came for healing for many years.

There has been a lot of illness in my family and I've had to deal with Type 1 diabetes since I was 18. Being diabetic also keeps me healthy – good diet, exercise – a diabetic's way of life is probably one that would benefit most people.

The Wednesday clinic fills me with peace. I can never work full-time in a normal 9 to 5 job now, because of my commitment to Wednesdays at the clinic. This has kept me sane and of course, slightly less well off, as I work part-time at jobs that keep me fulfilled and my soul happy. For me, meditation is the skill that I have learned that brings me most peace. Finding inner stillness once a day is the gift that allows me to keep going on my healing path.

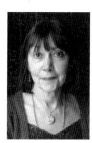

Cynthia Lomas

When I was a probationer for the College Accreditation Healers' Course in 1977, I worked with June (Frost), who was at that time the leader of the Monday healing clinic. I continued to work in the clinic when I was accredited, but left in 2000 when diagnosed with a heart problem caused by a virus.

In September 2005, I met June by chance at the college and she invited me to join her Wednesday clinic. I worked for about 18 months, then I had to leave because of work changes. In September 2007, I was diagnosed with heart failure. I am now retired and want to expand my healing work now that I have more time, and so I rejoined the clinic last year. It is a privilege to work in the Wednesday clinic; all the healers are very dedicated and June is my ongoing mentor.

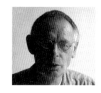

Thomas Nall

I don't honestly know how I got into this healing stuff. I didn't go searching for it or anything. I had stopped drinking for about a year by then and I wasn't looking for anything but maybe wondering what I should do next. I do remember that I was in a garden. Suddenly I just thought to myself 'Perhaps I ought to get more spiritual'.

It was odd because everything started happening after that. I kept meeting people who were interested in it, even at work. A woman came to my work, a healer. I was really cynical about it all and told her 'I don't believe in it'. She gave me some healing and the rest is history.

Aoife Nally (receptionist)

I have had many healings before of many modalities; Reiki, sound, cystal, prayer ... you name it. I had even trained in Magnified Healing, as far as the third phase. I had fallen into a deep depression, which led to a feeling of paralysis, many nights of insomnia and a stomach ulcer. Most days I felt crippled and crushed by the weight of life.

One morning I had a dream I should come to the

College of Psychic Studies and volunteer for any job going. Happily, they were seeking a receptionist for the contact healing clinic. This gave a very helpful shape to my week. I'm not sure if it was the people, the routine or the healing itself but every Thursday ... the day after the clinic I could function ... All the worldly things that stressed me out before were manageable. I found I was suffering less panic attacks and sleep was attainable.

Having experienced one-to-one healing, I have to say, group healing had a lot more 'staying power'. I am very grateful.

Oonagh Newman

I joined the clinic at Easter time in 2007 as a student at the College of Psychic Studies. At that time, I was waiting to undergo major surgery, which occurred during the summer of that year. I received healing prior to and during the immediate post-operative period and made a full and speedy recovery. I was in hospital less than 48 hours instead of a week and felt well enough to return to work within a month, not the 3 months suggested by the medical team. I attribute this to both the contact and distance healing given to me.

Many of my friends and colleagues, who are unable to attend the clinic, ask to have their names and names of family and friends added to the distance healing offered.

Valerie Renaud

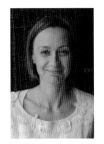

I actually joined the Clinic a long time after I'd finished my training at the College. I took the course for myself and that was the end of it. I was working at EMI at the time, a very busy environment and thought that that was me: a very busy person, always doing things! But then I quit and tried to find a job but couldn't find anything that was appealing to me: it was missing something but I couldn't figure out what. Then I went to the beach and was standing there looking at the waves and there it came to me: I had to be a healer.

And so I decided to join the clinic and I think it's just

fantastic to give healing to all these people who, like me, need healing, and can find it at the clinic. They know they can find love, care and light but no judgement. It's also nice to meet other healers who can share their experience. I just love it!

Kathy Schwadlak von Muller

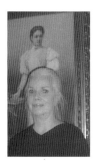

Kathy standing in front of the portrait in the healing clinic of Elizabeth Hope. She was a medium who used the name Madame d'Esperance. There is a full colour portrait in the Colour Section.

My journey into healing began in 1977. I was going through an intense period of pushing myself 24/7 with the intent of transforming my artistic skills into an art form that could provide me with a decent income. After much struggling and disappointments in trying to create "good art" (whatever that means!), I "let go" and gave myself permission to do "bad art". What I came to experience was a dramatic shift in my consciousness which included a great sense of well-being, an ability to connect with information and materials and a greatly enhanced creativity. I found myself very pleased with my artistic and financial results.

Having gone through hell to get to this state, I came to wonder if there could have been some easier way to achieve this. Three days later, I was browsing in the magazine section of Selfridges and I came across an article in "Psychology Today" about bio-feedback training and expanded states of awareness. This was a real "Eureka" moment. I was soon enrolled in what was to be the first of many courses over the ensuing eight year period, until the death of my mentor: Maxwell Cade[*6], a pioneer in bio-feedback training. The first thing I discovered was that I was indeed experiencing a distinct creative state.

I was to go on to explore healing, Zen, psychic realms and much more. The Maxwell Cade Foundation, started after his death, continues to expand his extraordinary body of research and training. In 1979, two books came out which were to profoundly shape my life and indeed continue to do so. One being Max Cade: "The Awakened Mind – Biofeedback and the Development of Higher States of Awareness" and the other written by a medical doctor and healer: W. Brugh Joy: "Joy's Way – A Map for the Transformational Journey – An Introduction to the Potential for Healing with Body Energies." 11 years later Brugh Joy published "Avalanche- Heretical Reflections on the Dark and the Light" an exploration of humanity in all its richness and complexity.

What I now realise is that my original decision to "let go" i.e. relax was to be the key, the "precondition", "the bottom line to altering many seemingly unrelated conditions or states. Relaxation is most important for good health as well as to access meditative, healing, creative and other states of expanded consciousness. Based on my own and my clients experience I have found that the simplest and most versatile technique for relaxation is breath control which has three distinct phases; that is (1) inhaling to a count, (2) holding ones breath to a count and (3) exhaling to a count. Max Cade was taught a version of this technique as a child to practice as he walked: 4 paces in-breath, 10 paces holding his breath and 6 paces to exhale … a great idea for an energetic child. One may try different counts.

Breathing through the nose and out through the mouth seem to enhance the relaxation process. Breath control can fit in anybody's life. It can be practised almost anywhere: at the computer, washing dishes, sitting in the bus … and so on. Taking the first step in breath control may reveal a path that may delight and surprise.

Maria Spellar

Initially I joined the healing clinic as a receptionist, although at that time I was in the second year of my training as a healer. Once passing the accreditation, I was offered the chance to join and work with the other healers in the contact healing group.

My reason for becoming a healer was quite by chance; I was encouraged to train as a healer while working as a co-ordinator in a stroke group in West London. My husband had a severe stroke, which left him severely incapacitated, and I naturally became his carer. His

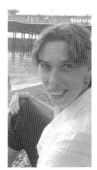

Maria on a trip to Brighton (the pier in the background) to interview Ray Brown and Paul in September 2009

recovery process took between 3 and 4 years, and he was in and out of hospital regularly.

Throughout that time, I became the co-ordinator of the West London Stroke Group, where I worked for over 3 years. I was interested in the healing process so I invited 2 healers from UK Healers (http://www.ukhealers.info/) to come to the stroke group to give some therapeutic support. I felt the members of the stroke group would benefit from healing. I immediately noticed the difference in the members after several weeks. They became more enthusiastic and motivated in helping themselves to cope with their disabilities, as well as providing them with a sense of peace and calm to their well-being. This fascinated me and I decided to enrol on the healing course.

Mya Stevens

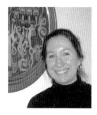

I joined the clinic to get experience in a practical sense, also to meet other healers and learn from their expertise.

I do have experience with mental health problems, as do many people I know (e.g. depression, anxiety). I've also worked for a disability charity for the past 2.5 years, so I know what it's like to live with illness and disability on many levels.

I think the clinic is great - it gives valuable practice to healers just starting out, and shows how lovely the regular healers are that attend every week, volunteering their time and energy for free!

Lon Teija

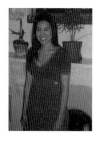

I have so much joy in my soul and I wish to share it by helping people. The healing clinic welcomes all those who embrace healing and are in need of extra support and encouragement.

I joined because I love being a part of the healing community and the personal healing journeys of others.

Cherina Tully (receptionist)

I came to the College of Psychic Studies after viewing their vacancy for a voluntary receptionist for Wednesday's healing group. Since being here I have had the privilege to witness the difference healing can have on a person. I see it in their faces as they come out from a session. They positively glow! I know first-hand how powerful healing can be and I hope we can raise even more awareness for this therapy and its healers.

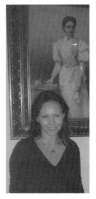

 Testimonials from healees about healing
"You've made me feel so strong. I feel more myself"

"It's changed my life. It's so powerful."

Cherina Tully

"I feel so relaxed; I could stay here forever. Thank you."

"I have had a very good week. I slept better and I've used the meditation you suggested. I feel more in control."

"I need to tell you this. This healing is changing me. Even my partner has noticed the difference. He says I'm happier, more content."

"My tumour has shrunk to 50%."

"There's really something in it. My specialist said 'I don't know what you're doing but whatever it is, keep it up.' I asked her if she believed in comple mentary therapies. She doesn't.'

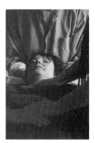

Tracy Hepworth
I have been using the Group Healing Clinic at the College of Psychic Studies since January 2008, when I was diagnosed with breast cancer. I have attended both the Group Healing sessions and separate One to One healing sessions. I believe that the healing I have complements the traditional medical treatment I am receiving.
    Although I am lucky that I have no major side effects

Tracy at the group healing clinic in the college in July 2009.

117

from the treatment, the energy boost that I receive from the healing has enabled me to remain active and to carry on as normal a life as possible. I have continued to work during my treatment. The energy boost that I receive from the healing helps me to work full time without any restrictions. My boss could always tell when I'd been for healing as he commented that I bounced back in the office, more energised than when I left. My treatment continues to be successful and I have found having a positive attitude has helped me considerably in dealing with my condition and the treatment.

Anna Wells

Anna Wells with Ray Brown in the background at his clinic in Hainault in August 2009

I sometimes had backache but it never really interfered with my day to day life - after all, I had no time to dwell on my niggles with a family to raise and a full time job to do. Not to mention a full social programme! Then it struck, really bad lower backache which progressed to full blown sciatica and ended with complete numbness in my right leg. I was really, really frightened!

A swift referral to a spinal consultant surgeon was made and after the usual diagnostic procedures, I was informed that I had a severe Spondylolisthesis. This is a condition of a defect in the vertebrae, in which they slip forward causing the spinal nerves to become distorted. The only hope of a permanent cure was an operation to fuse the vertebrae and insert rods to stabilise the condition.

The consultant gave the impression of a "run of the mill" op. I would be in hospital for about 4 days. I was still there a month later. My right leg was paralysed and I had severe foot drop, which meant I couldn't walk and I was on strong medication for the pain. I was at such a low ebb I would have been happy to leave this world behind, if only I could! To cut a very long story short, after physio and even more painkillers I was told that nothing more could be done for me. I felt a total medical reject. Then by chance I met Sue, an old work colleague. Sue was horrified by my plight and she suggested I get in touch with Ray Brown. I ignored her advice at first as I was somewhat cynical and struggled on in agony. By now, with the help of a leg brace, I should have been able to walk a bit, but because of severe pain in my right side, I just couldn't. So, I thought "What have I got to lose!"

When I visited Ray, he knew exactly where the problem lay. He went straight to my lower back and he somehow released the sciatic nerve. The effect was almost immediate and the pain in my side disappeared as if by magic! I would say to anyone suffering long term illness or any 'hopeless case' DO NOT GIVE UP! At least not 'til you've seen this remarkable man; then you will not look back!

Win Gibbons

I went to the healing clinic at the college with my two friends, Pat and Gordian. We went by train and arrived at the College at about 11.30 or so. I was very impressed with the building. I love those old Georgian fronted houses with lots of floors and a basement. I was also intrigued I must say, to have a healing session that only lasted for 4 minutes. I was eager to know how it worked, having been used to healing sessions of half an hour or so and felt I wouldn't be getting my money's worth if it was any shorter. I was asked to fill in a form and then sat in the waiting room to be called. I was ushered into a larger room that was divided by screens and was shown into an area where three people were waiting for me around a couch. I lay on the couch with one

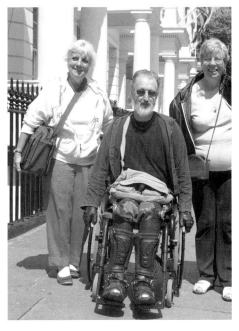

From left to right: Pat, Gordian and Win outside the College of Psychic Studies in July 2009

healer at my head, who tucked his hands under the back of my head. Another healer placed her hands across my chest area, another placed her hands across my sacrum area. I was told that an alarm was set and that it would go off when the four minutes was up. During the session I felt calmness and being used to complete relaxation techniques, I used these in conjunction with the healing. I can't say that I felt anything unique happening but I enjoyed the feeling of being relaxed and able to leave my body in the hands of the healers.

After the session they advised me to sit on the side of the couch until I felt 'grounded'. I was asked to select a drink from a collection of coloured plastic mugs, which I recognised as being the colours of the chakras. I chose a blue colour, which I was told, was the throat chakra. In all, I enjoyed the experience but didn't enjoy the journey.

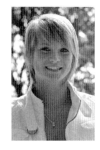

Kelly Patrick

Kelly has had health problems with her knee, her wrists and her back. Her first visit to see Ray Brown for healing was because of her knee. She'd had an operation and it left her with a lot of pain and also a kind of 'clicking' in the knee cap. She arrived to see Ray Brown on crutches several years ago. Kelly and I met at his Brighton clinic in September 2009.

"It was amazing. After the healing, I just walked out of the clinic." Now Kelly goes to see Paul for a yearly 'check up' but the knee pain hasn't returned. She has become part of the White Dove Spiritual Healing Group in Battle working as a healer with her mother, Reverend Debbie Thomas of the International Church and Healing Fellowship (ICHF).

Pat Cooper (pic opposite)

I have never experienced anything quite like it. I laid on the couch (in the Group Healing Clinic in the College) and three ladies asked me questions about my medical problems, if I had any. Luckily I am in good health but I still had the healing. I really had what can only be described as an electric shock pass right through me. So much so, that I felt somewhat strange after this session, and actually had to be helped from the couch.

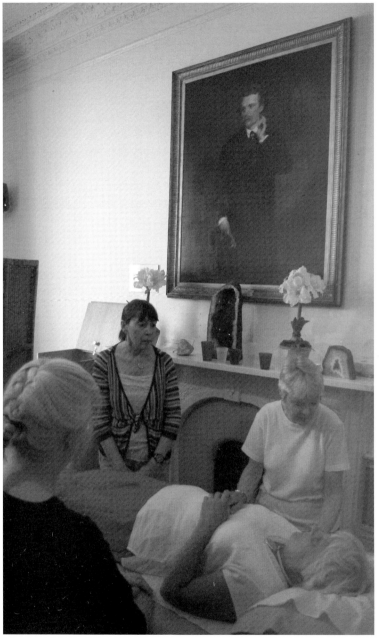

Pat Cooper from our creative group on the couch discussing her experience with the healers at the clinic in the College of Psychic Studies in July 2009. The portrait is of a college medium, Daniel Dunglas Home

It was amazing. Subsequently, I described it as 'a Damascus moment' in a later art workshop with the group.

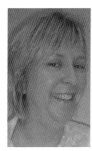

Beverley Evans

I have had the chance to experience healing sessions for myself but my real comments have to be about the healing sessions I witnessed at my school. These young people experience social, emotional and behavioural difficulties and are usually tense, loud and unable to relax, listen to others or communicate.

I, and my colleagues, were amazed as we witnessed our students engage and respond to the healing in ways we might never have imagined. Facial expressions completely changed. One young man on the autistic spectrum (ASD) came out and was not only calm and relaxed but smiling, something he rarely does and the next day he reported to going home and sleeping. His mother could not believe it.

Other students reported feeling electricity and some were able to verbalise feelings and emotions around anger in a very descriptive and informative way.

My own experience with healing is quite a strong physical reaction. Initially, as I sit upright and calm, I feel nauseous and dizzy almost like my body resisting to it and I have to fight to make myself absorb the calm and peace. I find the experience intense and completely worthwhile.

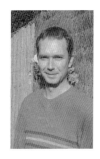

Tino Schroeter

My name is Tino and I attended a 15 minutes healing clinic session with a team of 3 spiritual healers, (as a volunteer as part of the project with people with longterm illness). Fortunately, I haven't got a medical history or any other difficulties at the moment. I attended the healing clinic just with the intention to get in contact with spiritual healing methods, to look how it works and what I can feel during the session. It was a great feeling to enjoy the warm atmosphere, to be surrounded by monotonous music, to listen to smooth voices and to feel warm hands on your body. After the session, I can't deny that I was more relaxed than before.

But to be honest, something must be wrong to feel not

relaxed under such conditions. I think it is definitely an excellent method with a positive effect. In my opinion, spiritual healing methods cannot replace conventional medicine but they can support the important link between body and mind. There is no harm in trying.

Julia Cotton

I have been attending the clinic for a good few weeks - I have had some long term physical and emotional issues dating back to when I was six months old ... (I am now 46) and I came to the clinic with the hope that the healing would help me with these very old issues and assist me on my spiritual journey. Well it has surely helped me in so many ways, ones which i did not expect and those I did expect (hope for).

I feel calm and centred when I leave the clinic and whilst I am there you all take such good care of us all, it really really is and has been a pleasure coming along. We are truly blessed having the clinic.......

Many many thanks.

Notes

[*1] Dolores Krieger, Therapeutic Touch, published by Piatkus

[*2] The seven levels of healing, Lilla Bek and Philippa Pullar

[*3] Auras - the energy field which surrounds the body. See Chapter 4 for full discussion

[*4] Ray Brown, spiritual healer. See Chapter 2 for an interview with him.

[*5] NFSH is the National Federation of Spiritual Healers

[*6] Researcher Maxwell Cade, who won a research grant from the College. See Chapter 4 for full discussion.

Aura photography

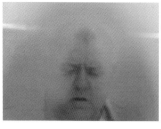
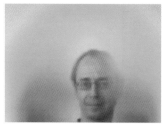

Far left from the top:
1. Charlie, resting aura
2. Aura before healing.
3 and 4. During spiritual healing
5. Afterwards

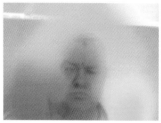
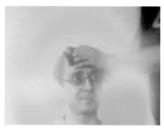
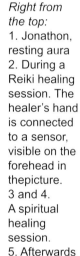

Right from the top:
1. Jonathon, resting aura
2. During a Reiki healing session. The healer's hand is connected to a sensor, visible on the forehead in thepicture.
3 and 4. A spiritual healing session.
5. Afterwards

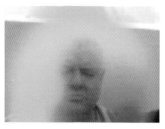
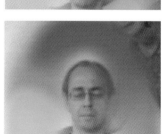
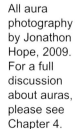

All aura photography by Jonathon Hope, 2009. For a full discussion about auras, please see Chapter 4.

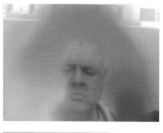
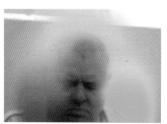
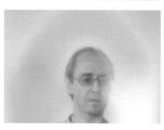

125

Aura photography

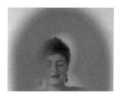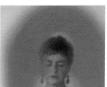

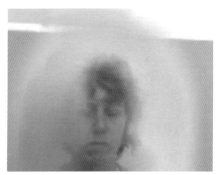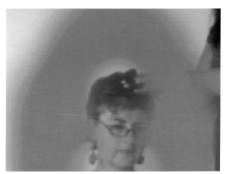

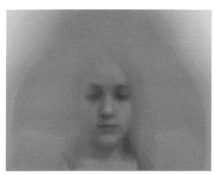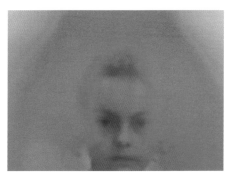

Above from the top:
1. Lizz Daniels
2. Lilu, aged 7,
   Lizz's
   grand daughter

Right::
Jonathon explains
to Jesscia while
Lily watches.

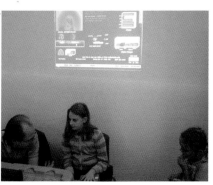

Above from the top:
Tina Lawlor Mottram;
1. Resting aura
2. During meditation
3. Reiki healing during aura
   photography, showing
   more orange in the aura
4. Lily, aged 8, Tina's
   daughter

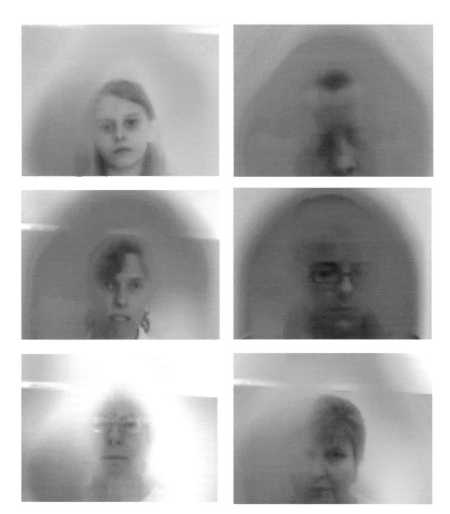

Above from the top:
The Spellar family
1. Jessica, aged 9
2. Her mother Maria

Below
3. Win Gibbons

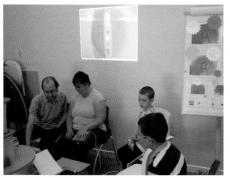

Above from the top:
The Ward family
1. Keiran, aged 8
2. Nathan aged 12
3. Their mother,
    Jane Ward

Left:
Jane with her hand
on the sensor, while
the family watch on

Art by
James Solly

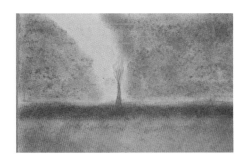

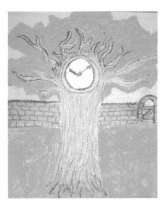

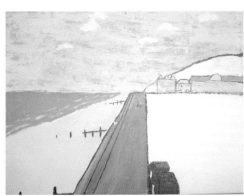

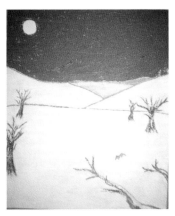

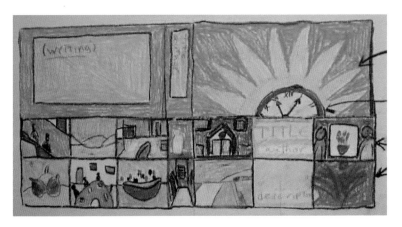

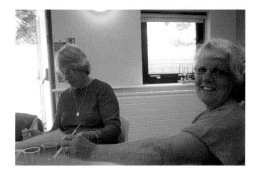

Win Gibbons (left) and Pat Cooper (right) painting, and meditating in our room at Sunlight. The garden can be seen in the background.

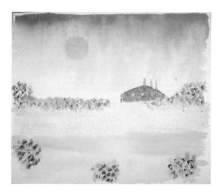

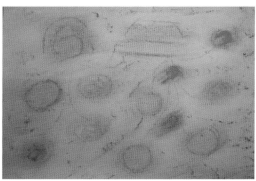

Above:
Art by Win Gibbons

Left:
Pat Cooper's masterpiece!

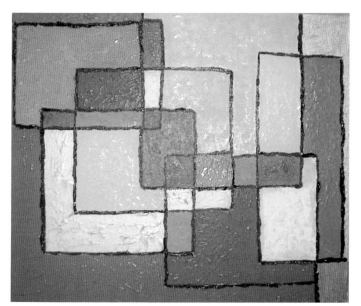

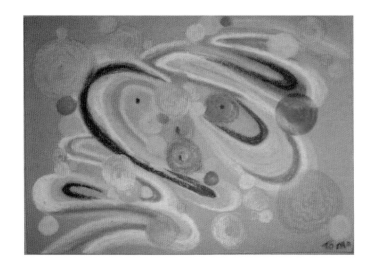

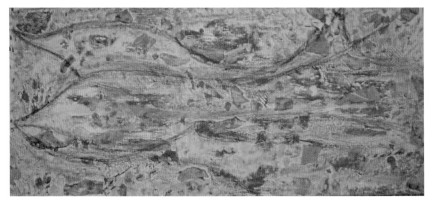

Art by
1. Tania
2. Lizz Daniels
3. Charles
Pankhurst

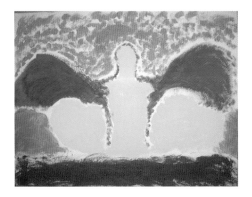

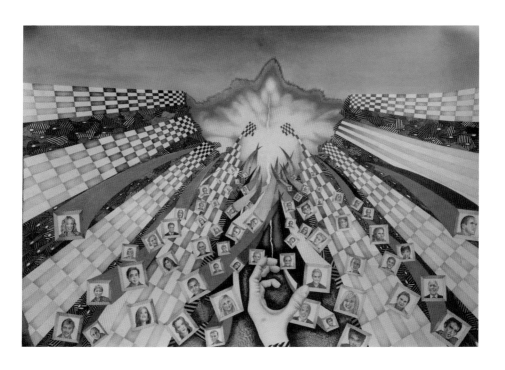

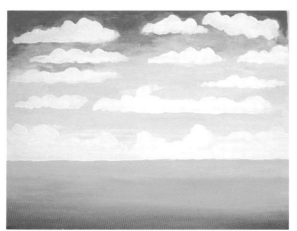

Above:
1. 9/11 by Ken Hopper
2. Clouds
3. Ken

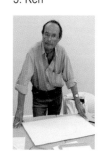

From the top:
Art by:
1. Lily Lawlor
Mottram
2. Gill Solly
3. Gill Solly

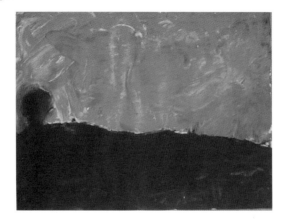

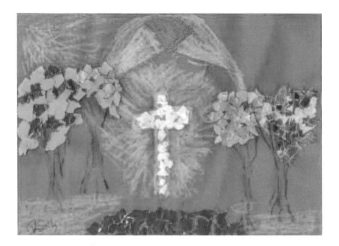

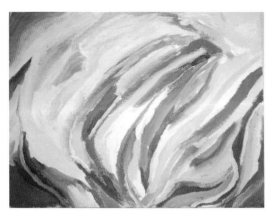

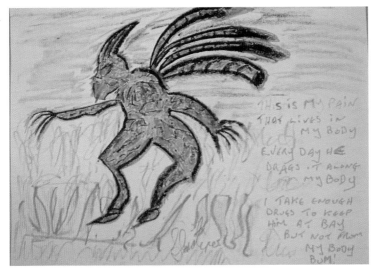

Art by
Gordian Bailey

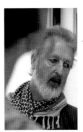

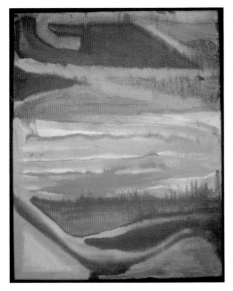

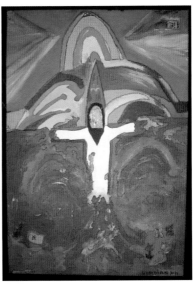

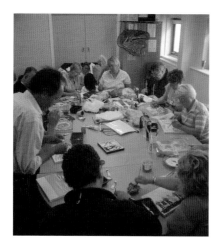
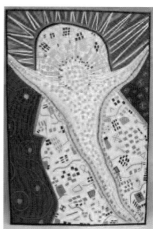
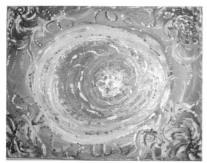
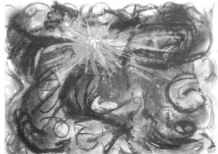

From top left:
1. The group at work
2. Angel by Lizz Daniels
3.4. Art by Lizz Daniels
5. Lizz Daniels holding 'A Burst of Joy'

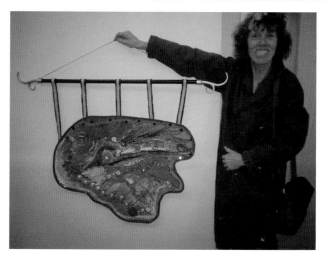

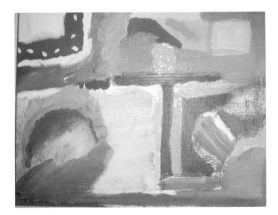

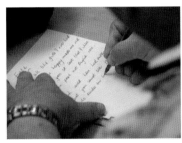

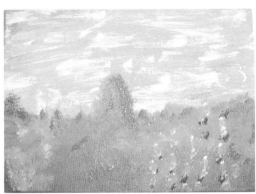

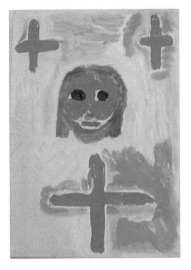

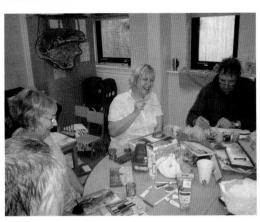

Above left
from top:
1. Beverley's art
2. Deirdre's art
3. Left: Charlie,
Deirdre, Beverley
and Doug

Above from top:
1. Charlie writing
2. Charlie's art.

Art from the top:
1. Derrick Solly
2. Rose Pope
3. Derrick Solly

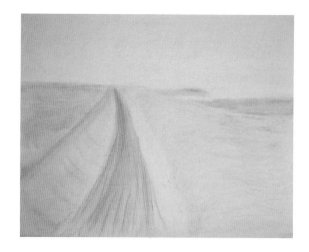

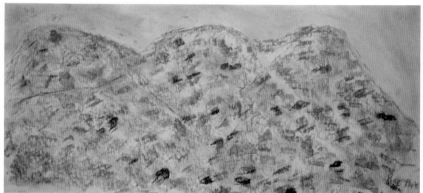

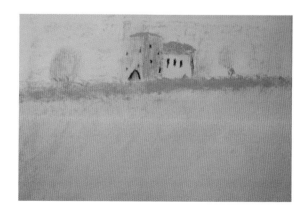

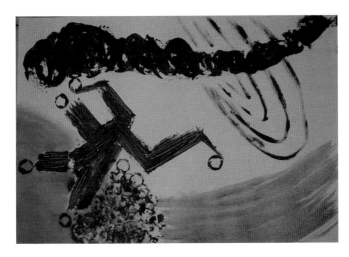

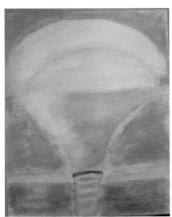

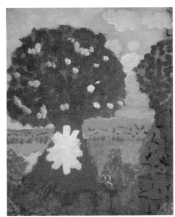

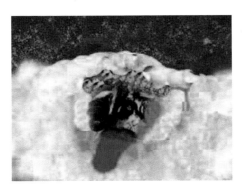

Art from the top:
1. Doug Fry
2. Doug Fry
3. Gill Solly
4. Doug Fry

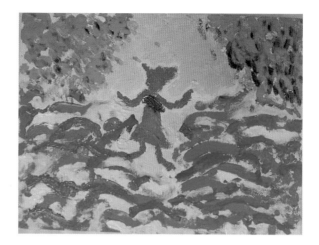

Art by:
1. Sarah Jenkin
2. Tina Lawlor
   Mottram
3. Sarah Jenkin
4. Gill Solly

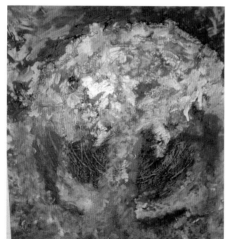

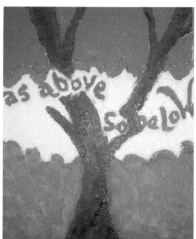

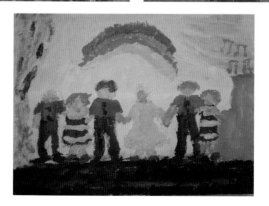

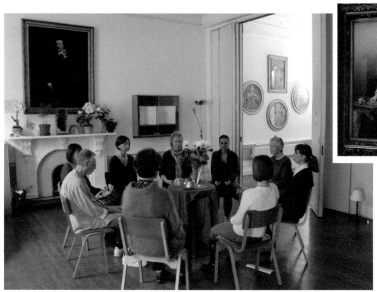

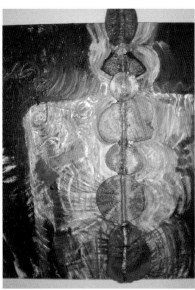

Above:
1. Elizabeth
Hope, Mme
d'Esperance
From left:
2. Meditation
for healers
3.4. Chakras
Tina Lawlor
Mottram

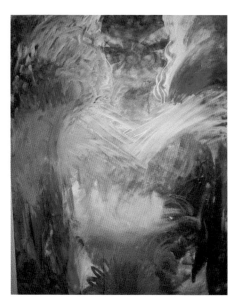

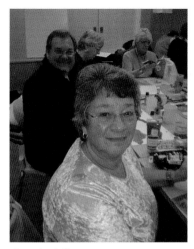
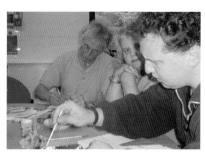
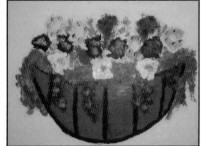

Above from top left:
1. Roy and Ann Moxon. 2. The Sollys
3. Ann's flowers. 4. Derrick's collage.
 5. Cerys Evans, with Deirdre.
6. Roy's Clouds

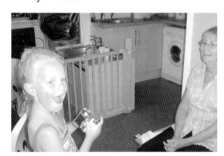
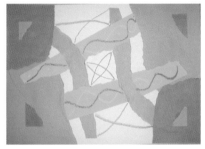

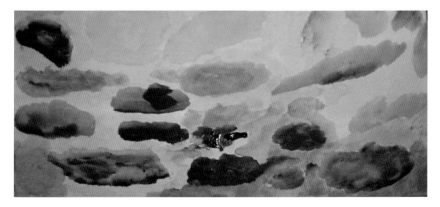

Chapter 4
The aura, meditation,
finding silence &
scientific research

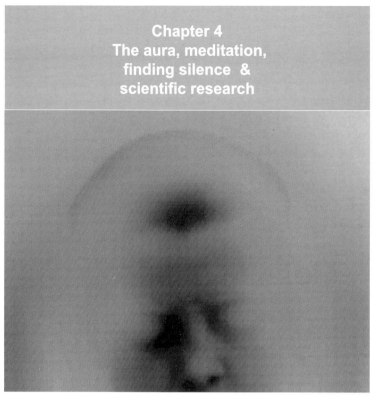

Keiran's aura taken in August 2009 at Sunlight. This can be seen in the Colour Section. *Photography by Jonathon Hope*

*"I believe we create our own reality – when I first
started coming to this group, I wondered what I
would get from it. Something had made me come.
We all talked about our illness and I thought perhaps
that's what it would always be – dwelling on
an illness. We pushed through the blaming and
moaning and whingeing and whining and
came through into something else.
Resistance was strong – we liked our illnesses
but the creative spirit was strong too.
What joy we had sploshing our paint on.
People smiled, the atmosphere was
charged with something other than sorrow.
ART is wonderful. Art can take us into
unknown territory. Wonderful stuff."*
Lizz Daniels

We have already explored the long term medical conditions of the people in our creative group, from a discussion of the conditions, through to the art and writing created on the project and some of the insights possible when working in ways alongside conventional medicine and using techniques not necessarily accepted by them. This chapter looks at the many ways to observe the human body, mind and spirit and also to record the experiences of the group as they explored these themes, related to their illness, health, spirituality and well-being. We look at meditation, reading auras, and how the scientists have been observing these states for many years. Maxwell Cade, who was twice awarded the Oliver Lodge Research Grant from the College of Psychic Studies, explored Biofeedback; the science of listening to the body and using the results to help the mind to control the body. 'The Awakened Mind'[N1] by Maxwell Cade and Nona Coxhead is a must for anybody looking for interesting research about the effects of meditation, spiritual healing, states of consciousness and scientific feedback about these processes on the human body. Cade and Coxhead promoted and experimented with the use of meditation, as they believed it is made more effective by combining meditation with Biofeedback. They describe the benefits of the art of meditation in great detail in chapter 3 of 'The Awakened Mind'. This provides a really in-depth exploration of meditation, its effects on the body and how it relates to Biofeedback. Stated benefits include:

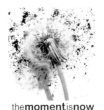

themomentisnow

• a decrease in oxygen consumption
• a reduction in carbon dioxide elimination
• a reduction in heart rate, respiratory rate, blood pressure, blood lactate, muscle tone and blood cortisone levels
• an increase was noted in perfusion of internal organs ie perfuse finger temperature and
• an increase in apparent basal skin resistance, which can be used as an accurate measure of the extent of relaxation

Most people are familiar with the well known 'fight-or-flight' response, that which causes a run of adrenaline in the system as a response to danger eg if a pot of boiling water is about to fall on a small child or they are about to put their hand into a naked flame, most people would rush to try to stop this happening. The hormone adrenaline is released in order to enable the person to do something out of the ordinary – a one-off response to danger or a threat. Adrenaline increases the strength and rate of the heartbeat and raises the blood pressure. It also speeds up the conversion of glycogen into glucose, which provides energy to the muscles. The opposite of this heightened state is the "relaxation response"; technically the 'trophotrophic response'.

Eastern cultures have long been aware of the benefits of meditation on the body and many Western doctors and researchers believe in its effectiveness as an aid to good health. Bernie Siegel [N2], is the doctor, surgeon and author who set up ECaP (Exceptional Cancer Patients) in the States. In his bestseller 'Love, Medicine and Miracles' he states that regular meditation tends to lower or normalise blood pressure, pulse rate, and the levels of stress hormones in the blood. Changes in brainwave patterns, something noted by Cade and Coxhead and many other researchers, are also noticeable. Meditation raises one's pain threshold and reduces one's biological age. Scientists and researchers agree that regular meditation is good for one's health, usually leading to changes in attitudes as well as physical health, enabling people to live better and longer.

The brain wave changes also lead to another major characteristic of the higher states of consciousness, namely the complete change which takes place in our sense of time, both in the timeless interval of the experi-ence itself and in an altered attitude to time thereafter. Cade and Coxhead postulate that during meditation, one's level of awareness is being changed, both of external reality and of oneself.

Meditation with our creative group

Gill Solly and her husband Derrick had a simultaneous image present itself to both in the group's first guided meditation. The atmosphere in the room was electric, no other way to describe it. Many people had never tried meditation before and this added to the excitement afterwards. Our creative group had just met for the first time. They verbally discussed their medical symptoms, diagnosis, medication, difficulties and effects on their lifestyles for over an hour, and then we simply sat for a few moments in complete silence, apart from the voice leading the meditation. Deep breaths inhaled and exhaled, a lifting from the ordinary into a simple place, alone with oneself for a few moments, allowing the body to relax.

For Gill, it was a place with trees, which became a symbol for her healing from breast cancer, later proved correct. Her husband Derrick also visualised this image and they were incredibly surprised at how this might have happened simultaneously. Gill says she had a vision of healing, with the tree at first representing the growth of the cancer. She found herself in her church all alone. Gill says she found it to be a lovely, warm feeling and she felt very safe and secure. She saw a coffin, pictured below, at the bottom of the picture. It had no flowers, no plaque, although Gill admits now that she thought it was for her. In front of this, Gill saw a huge old wooden cross, as tall as a man. She could see the stained glass window at the

Gill's Trees, created as a result of an image that came in meditation. They became a symbol for her recovery.

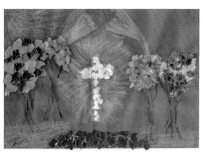

left hand side of her picture, which she later identified as the same side as her cancer. The cross was covered with white flowers. At first, as Gill watched, the flowers grew and grew until they completely covered the wood. Then a man with a beautiful face came to her, dressed in a silk cloak, which he wrapped around Gill's neck. Gill was comforted by the man who told her that she would be fine. After this she saw the treatment working and the tree went through spring, summer autumn and winter. Gill says when she looked back down the aisle of the church, the coffin had disappeared.

The image of the tree for both Gill and Derrick allowed them some peace when going to the hospital for results a few weeks later. Gill 'knew' she was getting better and the tests confirmed that her tumour had shrunk. Gill's trees can be seen in the collage she created on this project, showing the tree going through all seasons, emphasising the continual cycles of life and the spiral of growth and acceptance that comes with each stage of an illness and also its healing.

The group were encouraged to lead meditations too. The format of group meetings always started with hellos and introductions, followed by a meditation. It helped in what Lizz described as the social cohesiveness of the group in our project feedback notebook. 'The group is becoming more cohesive. Isolation and separation seem to be dissipating – good, friendly vibes. I remember when I first came how reticent everybody was. Now it's full on, hands in the paint, "let's get started" atmosphere. Throughout the session there were long periods of deep creative concentration.'

After meditation, the group then moved onto creative expression, having ensured that all the materials were available and to hand so that when eyes were opened, people could just start to depict or write what they had been through. There was some wonderful insight into the way the body can send intuitive messages to us, via meditation. Imagery seen in meditation can be useful to help people to recover from illness. Dr Bernie Siegel suggests that people should draw a picture of themselves, their condition or disease, and their treatment with their white cells eliminating the disease. An image showing how your body can heal itself and how it looks in the stage when it is healed, can be very helpful for people to look at how their unconscious is sending ideas, not necessarily in a linear, factual way.

Our creative group visualised their disease, illness or condition as an animal with some interesting results.

Sarah's response to one of the meditations is below. It contained the images that inspired her picture.

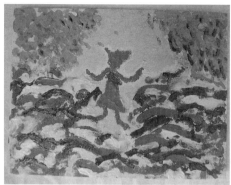

See this painting in colour on the cover.

"Honeybees, no room to move, everyone on best behaviour. The sea roars in my ears, what you call a miscommunication in my own body, doctor speak for "dunno mate". It's tinnitus that keeps me awake nights, not the doctors. It might be my body, but I don't have their training, do I? The seashell at my ear echoes back the rage when I am dismissed.

I feel it in my bones, when something is not right. I know my own body, cold and unresponsive as it is and I am ready armed with information. You do not fool me.

Take a deep breath, you say, think back to when you felt strong and well. The answer is already there, whispering in my ear.

Untameable and fierce, a restless energy never confined by convention or making nice. The sea moves to its own rhythm. I can be this, this is my strength.

When did I move to my own rhythm?

My body moving in time to the music, and I am gorgeous. My body shimmers with red glitter under the spotlights, and the audience roar approval. In burlesque baby, everyone is beautiful. All around other women, tall women, short women, thin and not so thin, reflect this glamour back at each other under the lights. Currents in my blood carry warmth to my limbs, my toes, my hips and

I   am   alive.

The disco zombie, back from the dead.

Later meditations with our creative group evoked the following responses in our feedback notebook:

• Enjoyed painting and relaxing with my new friends here. The visions of feelings and colour helped with the meditation. Deirdre.

- Through meditation, I saw the daffodil I did when I was a child and the music that lifts the spirit. There are things I can't do now. The small picture shows tossed salad and milk shake – a sign of my bad co-ordination now. Gill.
- The picture I painted was of a seafront. I enjoyed coming today. James.

Lizz was really excited by meditation and the way the group was changing.

- 'I believe we create our own reality. When I first started coming to this group, I really wondered what I would get from it. Something had made me come. We all talked about our illness and I thought perhaps that's what it would always be – dwelling on an illness. We pushed through the blaming and moaning and whingeing and whining and came through into something else. Resistance was strong – we liked our illnesses but the creative spirit was strong, Tina a great inspiration. What joy we had sploshing our paint on. People smiled, the atmosphere was charged with something other than sorrow. ART is wonderful. Art can take us into unknown territory. Wonderful stuff.'

Most people need to find their own way to meditate, as they do when trying to heal their body. The leader of this first guided meditation learned that not everybody can 'visualise' and that the way one person finds complete peace is not the same universal path. However, that said, the group have thoroughly enjoyed meditation as a group. We have worked with feeling unconditional love, in the way we feel about somebody on the planet and then trying to send that kind of love around the circle of meditation. The tangible difference in the room was a joy. People have been surprised at what insights come. For me, it is lovely to watch a group come together with compassion and to then create a piece of art or writing afterwards. "It's the highlight of my week" in the book just about summed it up for me!

Auras

According to Lilla Bek and Philippa Pullar[*3] in 'The seven levels of healing', the aura can be described as a protective electromagnetic field which surrounds the body. If you feel good in somebody's presence, they maintain, then it is likely they have a welcoming, large aura and people can relax into it and the person. In healthy auras, it appears to have a completely regular shape around the body. However, our energy fields also soak up atmosphere, from people, from places and no one is identical. On different days people will have different auras; we are all in constant change.

An aura is the energy field that surrounds the body, not visible to most human eyes. There are psychics and healers who can see them and healers work with this energy, often unable to see it but certainly sensitive to it. However, this ability to see auras is very rare. One person who can see them is Sue Allen, who works at the College of Psychic Studies. Sue works as a psychic, sensitive, healer, medical intuitive, psychotherapist, teacher and author.

She specialises in spirit release and psychic attack, clearing people and places of unwanted energies. Seeing the energy field around people who come to her for healing and spirit release is very useful. Sue describes the aura as an electromagnetic energy field, which surrounds the body and reflects subtle states, such as physical, emotional, mental and spiritual aspects. In a healthy person, Sue maintains that it is almost egg shaped, without dents or gaps. She also points out that the aura needs to be at a good distance from the body, to offer some protection. In a closed state this is about half a metre. "When a client comes to see me, I use 7 psychic senses to detect the aura: I feel it. Is it light? Is it vibrating? If so, at what speed? I look at its size, its shape, note if it has been dented and where this has happened. Is it complete? What colours can I see?" Sue describes the different layers, which exist in everybody's aura.
• The first is the etheric layer, which reflects the physical. Changes here can mean physical problems in the body.
• The second layer is the emotional layer, and here I see if there are emotions held in the aura, what colour they are and where they are stuck or blocked.

• The third layer is the mental layer, which shows what thoughts and beliefs the person has. Sometimes, certain thoughts are so frequent that they are apparent in the aura as thought forms.

• The fourth layer is the spiritual layer. Sue also checks the whole aura for spirit attachments, psychic attack, cords, past life events and karmic issues etc.

Sue has worked with many people with mental health issues and she can view certain patterns in auras of people with particular conditions. For example, imagine that the aura in a healthy person is like an egg shape. She scans the aura for mental health issues and for spirit attachment. Depressed people usually have grey patches in their auras, mainly around the head, and sometimes extending down the body. Sometimes the grey colour even reaches down to the feet, in severely depressed people. People with schizophrenia often have a split in the aura. "I have seen one starting at the lower back in the sacral area and rising upwards towards the head. Its shape was quite jagged, and it continued in a line until above the top of the head to the top of the aura." It seems that depression travels down and schizophrenia travels upwards. "For this person, I started working on the sacral area, trying to heal the issues, as this was where it had started."

We also discussed that it is noticeable that a group can sometimes have similar colours in their auras. "I used to lead the distant healing clinic and asked people to send love round the circle, sending to the person on the left and receiving from the right. This would create a red or pink, heart energy in people who took part in this exercise. Any close group can share energy and colours in this way."

Aura interpretation, like any process, is very dependent on each person reading it. Many books on the subject believe that certain colours determine *chakras* affected and so on. We have already seen in Chapter 2 that the earliest research by CW Leadbeater did not find the 'rainbow' of colours associated with *chakras*, as envisaged in current theory. Sue Allen does not think colours in the aura are fixed. They may mean something to one psychic or healer and not the same thing to another. When questioned about experiments done with groups of healers, Sue stated that most people, in aura workshops that she has taught, tend to see the predominant colour in an aura. There is generally a high level of agreement at the first observation but when people go into it in depth, they may all pick up different areas and colours and layers. This concurs with research carried out by Dr Daniel J Benor[*4], who asked 8 healers who were able to see auras, to describe the auras of people with known medical problems in a study in the UK in 1992.

Each healer was asked to draw a picture of the colours they saw around each patient. They also wrote down their interpretation, which they subsequently read out loud to the group. Many of the healers picked up completely different areas and colours. However, when revealed to the patients, they agreed that an aspect of their auras described by all the healers, bar one, resonated with them. This surprising result Dr Benor surmises, may be because healers pick up a selected part of the aura, not the whole visible image.

I asked Sue Allen about interpretation of auras. She stressed that auras reflect changes in us and that we change all the time, every day. A kind thought or a compliment paid will produce a very different aura to anger for example. The colour white in an aura often reflects a spiritual presence, usually a spiritual visitor. Purple tends to reflect somebody's spiritual intent or they may be using it to protect and hide some part of them. If the aura is very close to the crown, Sue says she would ask the person 'how do you feel?' as this type of aura can mean pressure on the crown and lead to headaches etc. The aura of somebody with Aspergers might cause an aura to be very close to the crown, for example. We also spoke about auras with colours inverted eg red at the crown and purple at the base/root *chakra*. (See page 69 for a fuller discussion about *chakras*) This could in rare cases mean that the whole auric field is inverted, which could cause many problems for the person was Sue's advice. Red around the head can show angry thoughts but can also indicate passion for example.

It is important to look at each individual. It has been shown that auras of people who have positive feelings to each other tend to move closer and merge. In sharp contrast, those who feel negatively towards each other find that their auras tend to retract from each other. We spoke about merging with other people's auric fields, while in our day-to-day travels, eg on public transport. Sue says that sometimes we may not like the mixing that happens, because we are used to our own energy and may feel that somebody else's is heavier or in some way unlike our own. Healers need to be conscious that this occurs, and ensure that protection is in place before healing takes place.

Sue says that she tends to divide auras into obvious zones for interpretation; the left side for her is the feminine aspect; the right side is the masculine. She believes that the aura at the back represents the past for the person and the front is related to the present and the future. She refines interpretation by looking at the layer an issue originates in and then proceeds with healing, and maybe questioning the healee about it.

If you are interested in learning how to read the aura, the easiest way to start is to look out a window on a sunny day and to watch trees is Sue's advice. The faint, 'jizzy' line is the etheric layer of the tree. We spoke briefly about experiments by Harry Oldfield and also the Kirlians who viewed the auras of plants, then removed a leaf then re-photographed the plant. The aura still showed the aura of this picked leaf still remaining on the plant! This was known as the 'phantom leaf' effect and was also explored with amputees. Jonathon Hope, our aura phtographer, talks about pain he used to feel from an amputated kidney later in this chapter.

Kirlian photography shows the energy field around the body

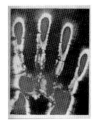

Aura Researchers

The term 'Kirlian' refers to a type of photograph called a photogram, made using photograph paper exposed with a high voltage. Semyon Kirlian worked on these photographic techniques in Russia with his wife, after discovering by accident that if objects are left on a photographic plate which is exposed to a high voltage, some surprising images are obtained. Small 'corona' are displayed, showing Kirlian claimed, the electrical field that surrounds objects. Likewise with humans, the Kirlians decided and worked on a series of images to show the energy field around humans, in their hands and all areas of the body. Their research released in the 1950s aroused a lot of interest and also some discussion about their view that the images shown could relate to the aura or human energy field that surrounds the body.

Other researchers continued the Kirlians' work and Thelma Moss made several trips to the Soviet Union to investigate this field. She worked at the University of California and after using psychedelic drugs, turned her attention to parapsychology including ESP, telepathy, hypnosis, ghosts. She worked and led UCLA's parapsychology laboratory in the 1970s. She explored a wide range of specific subjects in parapsychology (hypnosis, ghosts, levitation, alternative medicine), though her research on Kirlian photography was the most significant theme in her work.

Walter Kilner used special cyanin dyes on glass screens to induce auric vision. He reported that physical states correlate with auric changes. More recent explorations have refined these early observations. Harry Oldfield has built a Kirlian hand-gun, which fires high-frequency radio signals at the heart. Resonance of the heart is picked up by the gun and displayed on an oscilloscope, indicating anomalies. Dr Oldfield and Dr Peter Kandela have also photographed undiagnosed breast tumours in women.

Dora Kunz, a healer who worked with Shafika Karagulla, a neuropsychiatrist, to observe auras of patients, reported in 'The Chakras and the Human Energy Field' a study in 1989 that Kunz was able to provide information that closely correlated with the diagnoses made by Karagulla. There were also instances reported of Kunz discovering areas in the auras that showed a particular diagnosis, before it had been made by the specialist or any other professional. Well known healer and author, Barbara Ann Brennan, realised she could see tree auras as a child and later in adult life, she is able to use this ability to help people to recover from illness. Dr. Charles Tart, who worked at the University of California, noted that there appear to be four main types of aura: physical, psychological, psychical, and projected. Dr Tart also devised the 'doorway test' to investigate the aura. Next we move from the investigation of auras to a discussion of auras, by a member of our creative group.

Introduction to Auras by Jonathon Hope
Jonathon Hope's story can be seen in Chapter 1. He is a member of our creative group, who specialises in aura photography as an aid to healing.

An aura is the individual energy field that we all have around us. Much of my own personal understanding of this energy field comes simply from observation. Personally, I can't see auras. However, I use a device that can create a photo of our individual energy field called an `Auracam`. By using this I can help people understand the importance of their energetic body and work with them to rebalance and improve their mental, physical, emotional and spiritual self. This is based on the simple premise that when we better balance our mind, body and spiritual energies, we have the best hope of achieving a profound sense of well being.
Why did I buy an Auracam?
If a friend had mentioned five years ago that I would soon be buying a device capable of showing people's auras, I would probably have thought it ludicrous, or at best laughable. At that stage, as a person who was experiencing significant ill health, I had no idea whatsoever of the importance of our so-called energetic body or aura. I

153

wasn't interested in any therapies that worked through this subtle energy field. I had not heard of acupuncture, healing or reflexology. I was closed to the idea that my illness could be helped by anything but the scientific or medical approach that I had relied on for a quarter of a century. But here I am now, a short while later, using an Auracam to help people not just connect with the reality of their non-physical self, but also to gain deep, profound, personal insights into their emotional, physical and spiritual well being. So what happened?

Well, by chance I was thrust, quite unceremoniously, onto my own road to Damascus! It happened in late 2006 just after I started to study Egyptology at college, where I became intrigued by the mystery and antiquity of ancient Egypt. Shortly after, I arranged to join a small group travelling to Egypt for a few weeks. After arriving in Cairo, we set about trying the local food, visiting the Great Pyramid and exploring various temples and holy sites. I wasn't into religion or spirituality, so I just went along to gaze in wonder at the breathtaking architecture.

Whilst wandering the halls and chambers of the vast and incredibly well preserved temple complex at Dendera, I began to feel a familiar pain starting to radiate from my mid / upper back. This pain had started 4 years previously when my original kidneys had been taken out. I had labelled it phantom kidney pain after the so called 'phantom limb' phenomena experienced by amputees. At the time I knew that the pain would significantly worsen and immediately regretted leaving my most powerful painkillers on the boat. So I just gritted my teeth, carried on walking and tried to take my mind off it. After three hours or so, the pain became too overwhelming to hide, so, not caring that the rest of the group would wander off, I slumped down to rest, physically and emotionally drained.

After five minutes or so, the group leader asked me what was wrong, I explained about the pain and asking if she could try and help, she placed her hands about a foot away from my back. After about twelve minutes, the pain disappeared. A wave of relief, near euphoria swept through me. I was incredibly grateful, but at the same time, I couldn't quite believe it. Even strong, quasi opiate medicines couldn't take the pain away – they took the edge off, but nothing could remove it like that! I remember thinking to myself, whatever this is, why is it not available on the NHS? I was actually quite angry that it wasn't. She hadn't even touched me! I couldn't understand. How had she done that? Over the following three or four days on five separate occasions, this powerful pain was quickly taken away. After that it never came back. In fact, it has never come back to this day.

Eventually it was explained to me that the healing energy had come from the universe or source and had passed through her hands to my body via an energy field or `aura`. Though incredulous, I couldn't deny that something astonishing had happened. Then and there I vowed to understand what had happened to me and to explore this so-called energy field or aura, as well as the principles of healing itself. Because the logical, rational part of me couldn't simply take this concept on faith, that commitment eventually lead me to buy the Auracam. I wanted to see this so-called energy field myself, I wanted to measure it, observe it, explore it and understand it.

What is an aura?

An aura is a colourful electromagnetic egg-shaped energy field that surrounds us all. In fact, it surrounds all living things, including adults, children, dogs and horses. Adult auras tend to be dynamic and rich, ever-changing and with a huge variety of colours, each of which has a specific meaning. The colour or frequency of this energy field is an important clue in interpreting an Aura. Children tend to have lighter, more pastel shaded colours, often dominated by a presence of red, a colour that is usually associated with dynamic physical activity or excess energy! Once, whilst working with the Auracam overseas, a young girl asked her mum if she could see her own Aura. Hopeful, she asked "Do you think mine is pink?" Sure enough, when she put her hand on the plate, clouds of delicate, chrysanthemum pink coloured energy materialised around her head. We were speechless. Speechless, but as delighted as she was.

Many of us are used to seeing images of auras, though we may not know it! The paintings of the great saints, of Jesus and Mary, the sculptures of Buddha and the four thousand year old temple etchings of the Egyptian Gods often depict a so-called halo. Did they know something we didn't? Well the halo is simply the part of the aura around the head. Interestingly, the Great Masters of the Italian Renaissance painted the auras gold. How did they come by this information? Perhaps we will never know. But, intriguingly, this colour or energy around a spiritually enlightened person makes sense. Our first ever Auracam photo was of a young man struggling daily to bringing positivity, compassion, wisdom and spiritual insight into his day-to-day life as a City trader!

Edited up to hear

Our individual energy bubble is constantly changing, influenced by our actions and especially our thoughts and emotions. Indeed, each thought and emotion itself has a colour. Using the Auracam, it is possible to immediately pick up if a person is thinking or feeling a new emotion, because the colour of their aura promptly changes! However, in the medium term, there is also a `steady state`, whereby, for example, our aura colours may remain broadly similar for a number of months. When using an Auracam photo, this is the aura image that we try to capture. In time, a new energy will come in. Throughout our lives, there is this circulation of energy as our life path develops and our thoughts, emotions, experiences and attitudes change.

What is Aura photography?

Aura photography is the process of taking a picture of an Aura. It is believed to have started with Semyon Kirlian in 1939, who invented the first process to photograph the Aura, which showed what seemed to be a discharge of light round the edge of the hand. Since then, others have taken this process forward and the Auracam itself was developed by Guy Coggins in the US, who amongst other changes, added a camera and then a PC to capture the Aura in real time. This Auracam is the device I use and it visualises the aura and its component parts. In itself it is not a therapeutic tool. However, it can be used as a powerful tool to guide self transformation.

So why are auras so important?

Firstly, our auras depict our true inner self or our physical, mental and spiritual self. By using various techniques to work with our aura, we can better balance out our body, mind and spirit. When we do this, we can achieve a genuine sense of well being. So how might this work?

For example, for those of us who are predominantly logical, rational and analytical, this imbalance might be reflected in a greater vulnerability to stress and anxiety, our creativity may suffer, we may feel less able to tap into our intuition and relationships may be tougher. By rebalancing this mind based outlook, perhaps through occasional or regular meditation, visualisation or physical activity, we may experience a noticeable reduction in stress, a surge in creativity and problem solving abilities, a greater flow of inner-wisdom, a calmer mind and improved relationships.

Secondly, the colours of our aura show our energetic `toolkit` that is available to us at a particular point of time. By better understanding this toolkit, we can better manage our energy and focus on the most appropriate actions at that particular time. For example, the energy on the right side of our aura is what we use now, whilst the energy to our left is what we will use in the near future. Thus, if we have yellow energy to our right and red energy coming into the left, then now would be a great time to brainstorm a new project. However, implementing it, especially if it involves major physical activity, would best be delayed until the red energy is fully available for us to use.

Thirdly, our aura contains our seven so-called *chakras* or spinning wheels of energy. By balancing these *chakras* we can improve different areas of our body and our psyche. For example, we might see that our so-called base *chakra*, which is located near the coccyx or tail bone, is smaller than our other *chakras*. It might indicate that we have long standing concerns about our own safety and security, perhaps because of a lack of self confidence or because of prolonged health issues. Using different techniques, we can re-balance this aspect of our *chakras* so that we feel more confident, more grounded.

Fourthly, this energy field helps us understand our interactions with others. In other words, why we get on with some people and not with others. We have all experienced walking into a room and being drawn towards one person or another, even before we communicate with them! This is an example of our auras in action. For example, someone with a predominantly blue aura may be attracted to another person with the same colour aura, but not to another who has an orange aura. The former may, like him, be calm, open and easy going, but he may feel the latter's dynamic emotions, passion and energy to be outside his comfort zone.

Lily, aged 8, with Jonathon. Note her left hand on a blue handplate, which sends information to the PC and can be seen on the screen on the wall behind.

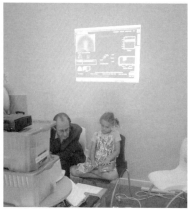

How is an Aura photo taken?

An Auracam is made up of a laptop, some pretty smart software, a webcam and a handplate. Working in concert, they pick up individual energy patterns, including the entire aura, the *chakras* and the overall Mind, Body, Spirit balance. The different frequencies of energy picked up by the handplate are translated into various colours and then superimposed around the webcam image.

What can you expect to see?

Aura colours emerge in an Auracam image like clouds around a picture of the person's face, some strong, some weak. Each colour provides insight into ourselves, each colour can mean something different from one person to the next. A predominantly red aura may mean that someone is either energised, confident, been out for a run, angry (hence the phrase `red in the face`) or simply passionate. For example, if one remembers a big bust up with the boss, then real-time, as that memory is recalled, the aura may shift to red. This illustrates the seemingly simple, but profoundly important insight that our thoughts and words have a very real, physical, tangible effect upon our own body. In one case, a mother's firm reminder to her young child not to remove her hand from the hand plate triggered an immediate flush of red through her child's aura.

Is there such a thing as a `bad aura?

In short, no. The aura tells us like it is. It gives us invaluable, objective feedback on our holistic well being. It tells us a little about our psyche, our emotions, our balance in life, framed in terms of our mind, body and spirit. It can help us understand our energy flow and how best to time certain activities. When having an Auracam reading, it is best not to have any preconceptions about a particular colour; we all need a mix of colours in our aura. For example, all of us needs a little red somewhere in our energetic body. It helps ground us. Keep us present so that we don't fly off with the fairies.

The importance of keeping an open mind is well illustrated by the case of a friend who was anxious about having an aura photo taken. She feared that she might have a particular colour in her aura that would symbolise something negative she was going through at the time. I explained that there was nothing to worry about and as she put her hand on the plate, a cloud of beautiful pastel rainbow - like colours emerged around her head. She relaxed and suddenly her aura went bright white! I was astonished. This was the first time I had seen this myself. I was just explaining this to the lady, when a person at the back of the room, who later explained that she could actually see auras, exclaimed: "Wow, did you see that? An Angel has just appeared at your right side!" Interestingly, a white aura usually signifies purity and truth. So an Auracam reading is never boring, but it rarely causes any fear!

Auras of our creative group

This project had set out to explore illness in creative ways and part of the project was the opportunity to see your aura. It had a profound effect on many people in the group, leading to confirmation of intuitive feelings and moving on with a greater understanding of their own personal traumas into the next phase of their lives. They say a picture speaks a thousand words and the reaction of the group was so positive to the whole experience that those who missed the day would really like to try it for themselves in the future. Both the images and the interpretation given by Jonathon seem to have given people a new perspective on their 'physical' body. Colour pictures of all the auras shown in black and white in the following pages can be seen in the Colour Section.

The person lays their hand on a handplate, which sends information to the computer, which then appears on a screen. This human face appearing on a projected screen, surrounded by colours that seem to shift shape, texture and intensity as the reading progresses was a magical moment for me in this project. I'm aware that I was quite nervous before I started because I thought nothing might show on the aura. How wrong can you be? As a healer, it seemed to 'prove' that what I know exists in the form of healing, heat and electrical tingling, magnetism or however it is described, actually does exist. There it was displayed before my eyes in glorious technicolour. I was also very interested to compare the adults' and children's auras in the group for any visual patterns linked to age, sex and perhaps family patterns.

As a trial before we worked with the group, Jonathon and I experimented with the equipment. We took some resting auras, and then tried some meditation and then healing to see if we could notice any effect on screen. We later repeated this experiment with Charlie in our creative group and the same result was very evident. Please see pages 125-127 for colour reproductions of these auras. On both occasions, when spiritual healing was given, a dark blueish indigo colour appeared on the screen. Naila

Hope is a Reiki healer and this healing, by contrast, showed onscreen as orange. It would be interesting to see if this is consistent with other healers or if it was a one off.

Tina Lawlor Mottram

For me seeing my colours on the Auracam was magical. I've worked with energy as a healer for so many years and can physically feel tingling, heat, cold and a strange type of magnetic, electrical sensation in my hands. However, I suppose on camera here was the 'proof' that I can never show people when they ask 'So what do you do when you heal?'. I could see a deep blue colour floating into Jonathon's aura and changing his aura too. Cade's research with Rose Gladden showed that she could alter the breathing and brain wave pattern of the healee. I know that this deep blue was not my aura colour, as mine had showed a vivid red and purple. I was very interested in the different colours that Reiki and spiritual healing show on camera too. This could be a future area of research for me. I had just cycled for an hour to get to this meeting and my energy centres were vibrant and very alive on screen. The whole experiment added a dimension to my healing; it allowed me to realise that all emotions register in our thoughts, in our auras and in our bodies in many levels.

This tool had an extra dimension for me. Jonathon states that the Auracam is not diagnostic and cannot be used as such. However, having visited my diabetic clinic a few weeks before this reading, I had been told that there was some suspicion that my kidney function was not as good as it might be. Nothing indicated this on my Auracam reading, which was quite a relief for me. Obviously, I would have to follow this up with routine blood and urine tests to confirm, but it was still comforting.

Overall, seeing the auras confirmed to me that the work I am doing with the group and in the healing clinic has a definite physical effect and that the aura camera actually provides me with a tool to show people what I 'do'. It has already been a valuable tool showing the proofs of the book to future clients, displaying the colours in the auras.

People, myself included, are excited, interested and intrigued about viewing their illness and their body in ways that offer new possibilities and hope.

I wanted to see if there were any family resemblances in auras and we had various groups included on this day - mothers and children, and a grandmother and grandchild for comparison. My child, Lily's aura showed as quite similar to her mother's. As she has no known health problems but is aware of her mother's, this was a great adventure for her. Jonathon's interpretation of her aura showed that mother and daughter have similar colours in the right; a violet colour, which is interpreted as 'an omen of benevolant supernatural ifluences or the joyous, highly spiritual energy you are putting out to the world'. There was a lot of red in both auras too, which can be inter-preted as passion, action, physical strength and 'intense activity'. Lily's had more orange than her mother's and this can mean 'originality and independence' and vitality, gregariousness and enthusiasm. Lily watched Jonathon very carefully indeed as he prepared and she seemd quite pleased about this interpretation.

Other families showed some similarities too. Maria Spellar's daughter echoed the same yellow in the right hand corner; the Ward family all showed pink in their auras. Jonathon explained to each person how colours in diferent areas could be interpreted. I had never seen white in an aura before and both Win and Lizz showed a floaty mix of pinks and whites. For both of them, this was quite a big discovery, as they describe below. The auras described on the following pages can all be seen in colour on pages 125-127.

Lizz Daniels
When Tina announced that we were going to have an aura cam session I was very excited. It was something I have wanted to do for years but because it's quite expen-sive I had always talked myself out of doing it. Now here it was being given to me as a gift. I had no idea of what the readout would be and this was a big part of the attraction.

It wouldn't be someone making a judgement of me but a machine registering my magnetic field and translating it into words that I could read. I felt I could really trust what came out of it and was a bit scared in case it was of a negative nature. No one was more surprised than me when Jonathon talked me through the outcome.

In fact I was bowled over, completely stunned by what he said. It was as if there was no denying my suppressed psychic gifts any more. It clearly stated in more ways than one that I held the power of healing within me and was very connected to spirit, in fact, Jonathon said that my readout was very unusual and that he had not come across such a strong sense of spirit in anyone before. Looking at the picture of myself, I could hardly believe it was me. It's not often one sees oneself with their eyes closed and I was very surprised to see such a serene looking person surrounded by violet white and gold colours. I do not consider myself serene and this was a wonderful affirmation about the self that is not visible. I meditate daily and have done since Rosie (Lizz's daughter) died but had never seen myself. It was truly a wonderful gift to see and has helped me to make steps forward in to realising other depths of my nature. I wasn't really able to read the printed paper until I was at home, for there was a lot to take in, but I found it very inspiring and uplifting.

Jonathon, who is also a medium, talked about what he saw and felt and suggested I went to see a fellow psychic at the College of Psychic Studies. A week or so later, I took his advice and booked myself an appointment, something I have never done before because of money. 'Spending money on myself is not easy. I need new teeth but can't get round to parting with cash to do it. Going on a workshop all day I can justify the cost, but for a one hour consultation…and the train fare!! But I did it.'

Since this moment, Lizz has assimilated the whole experience into a poem and moved on. She went back to study art at college and is invigorated by the whole experience. For Win, a crucial moment on this project was seeing her aura on screen. Here is her description.

Win Gibbons
I was aware of a tingling sensation in my left hand. When Jonathon told me my aura was pure white which indicates that I had angels present in my healing plane I could identify with this. I've had reason to believe that my son could be my spirit guide. He has been seen at a healing session I've attended. It confirms a lot of feelings I've had about myself. "When Jonathon told me that my aura was pure white, which indicates that I had angels present in my healing plane, I could identify with this. I've had reason to believe that my son could be my spirit guide. He has been seen at a healing session I've attended."

Charlie Wolf
'The remark about compassion and idealism is so true about me.' Tina Lawlor Mottram adds: We had a gap for a half an hour because somebody was delayed. There were 3 healers present so we decided not to waste the time and did some healing, both with Charlie and with Jonathon. For me, when the blue colour rushes in, it's a magical confirmation that the work we do is evident. The aura shifts suddenly and so dramatically; always this deep indigo blue comes with spiritual healing. The colour makes me so happy now when I see it anywhere else. I know that this colour for me has a special significance.

Maria Spellar (Jessica's mother)
I felt very relaxed. Jonathon explained very well. Significant details about my aura. Brilliant stuff!

Jane Ward (Nathan and Keiran's mother)
Very interesting experience. I knew a little about it and was interested in having it done. It's given me things to think about and focus on.

Nathan Ward
I found the experience very interesting and surprisingly,

most of it did sound like me and my main colour on the Auracam was red which is my favourite colour.

A last comment about the Auracam

Not even half the group managed to make the date scheduled for the aura photography. It has created a real stir in the group. As soon as people saw this etheric quality on a screen, it seemed to hit a nerve with so many people on the project. Everybody who was unable to attend is now very keen to attend any future session. The success of this part of the project speaks for itself. For me, any method that offers people with a longterm condition such hope, insight and pleasure must be seen as benefical and should be offered to people whenever possible.

NOTES

*1Cade and Coxhead describe the benefits of "the art of meditation" in Chapter 3 of "The Awakened Mind" p83-102.
*2 Bernie Siegel, author of 'Love Medicine and Miracles'
*3 Lilla Bek and Philippa Pullar, p54 'The seven levels of healing'
*4 Dr Daniel J Benor, who asked 8 healers to describe the auras of people with medical problems, known to the physician. 1992 study - 'intuitive diagnosis'. (Subtle energies). p399 Spiritual healing, Daniel J Benor. Healing Research, Volume I.
*5 David Furlong 'The Complete Healer'

Chapter 5
Trees, Poems and moving on

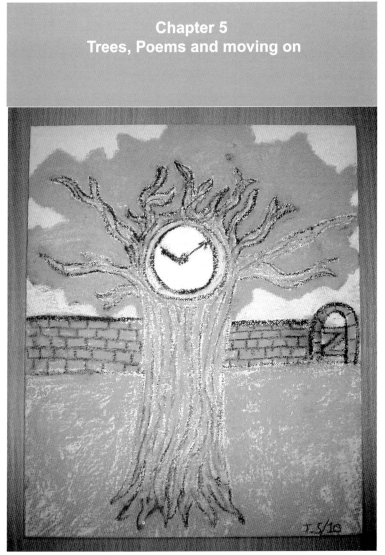

Tree
by James Solly
2010

There is no such thing as time.
There is only now.
Maxwell Cade and Nona Coxhead

the**moment**is**now**

Themomentisnow! works creatively with illness, using art and creative writing to explore themes. This book is the result of a project funded by Awards for All in 2009-10.

It is January 2010 and I ask the group if they would like the project to continue after the funding runs out. Most people are too busy painting or writing to comment but when I get the feedback sheets, I find wonderful comments by all. Ken Hopper gives his reasons: 'Yes, because I like to be involved.' The Solly family agree. 'Yes, as what we have learnt helps people help others.' Pat Cooper sums it all up in this comment: 'I really think that we have gelled as a group, and a greater under-standing of what other people have had to go through. We will keep in contact, and especially now that the website once fully operational, will play an important part in this endeavour because it will reach a much, much wider audience and can be regularly updated and used as a professional, and social tool to this end.'

What follows are the creative responses of people in the group, some themed on their illness and others giving reflections on life in general. Some people have been able to come to almost every session. Others have come when they can. For all of us, there has been some change and this is reflected in the poems, writing and paintings that follow.

My journey started with 'complications' of diabetes and during this year, I've discovered that my own intuition about my body is as valuable as a specialist's. I know that many others in this group agree with me. This makes us quite a powerful group. We recognise our need for medicine, information and doctors. However, we also define our right to be people, not NHS numbers. My specialist may not have given me a great diagnosis, but she has given me a great new line: 'This is the start of it now!' For me, *this* message is hopeful and when talking about humans, where there's life, there's hope.

In conclusion, I felt that Jonathon Hope's story was a fitting way to end this story of health; his advice is so uplifting and a story that could have had a bad ending. However, as the privileged story teller, my tale always has goodies and baddies, lots of adventures and inevitably a happy ending. Here's to a happy ever after!

Lightning Rod
Sarah Jenkin

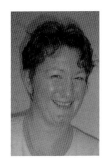

We need a place
To make a stand
and speak our
truth.

Take it or leave
it. Here is your
Permission.

Being a "good"
Girl doesn't
Deliver

The goods. It
Just makes
The paperwork
Easier.

The doctors do
Not know everything
And it is unfair
To expect them to
(Why do we assume
this?)

So come up.
Say something.
No one else will
say it for
You.

Insect Sarah Jenkin

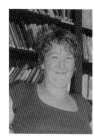

Self preservation; my shell is impervious,
a water-tight carapace. A fortress of
black, purples, reds
glinting a warning;
Stay back.
Infection oozes from every pore,
I am dis-eased.

Sometime Thursday afternoon, the
shell cracks;
beneath the ragged tear
fall circles of green, that caress, that
collide, that
console;
the gentle breeze parts the shadows,
a surprise of whiteness
burns a pattern onto my skin
of shade and dark mingled
with gold,

the breeze a memory
of ice-capped mountains,
drawing the itchy twigs together, a
standing ovation

my lungs greedily
gobbling, expanding to fill the sudden void;
impatient shoes dance away,
and
grasses fling
captured raindrops, a rapturous

baptism of dew

Dandelion;
a declaration by Sarah Jenkin
Inspired by my fight to reclaim my body,
even though other people didn't believe me

An orange signal-flare
explodes above splintered grass;
Crisp ambition glares out from
bellicose spikes; my
boundaries are clear and
sharp

themomentisnow

a brittle stalk, strong but light
braced securely above the sea of
gossamer ferns and bright-faced
impostors.
This is mine; within this circle,
my space, my
own

Lop off my head and another grows,
my roots are strong and reach far;
poison cannot hurt me, nor spades unearth,
my tongue defended by dent de lion,
the lion's teeth of Brighid;
Goddess of words, smithcraft and healing.
You will remember me.

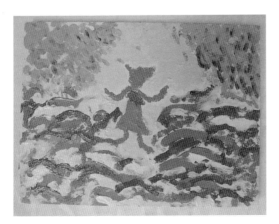

Doug Fry's story

Trigeminal Neuralgia (TN) is an extremely severe facial pain that tends to come and go unpredictably in sudden shock-like attacks. The pain is often described as stabbing, shooting, excruciating, burning, extremely strong. The pain usually lasts for a few seconds, but there can be many bursts of pain in quick succession. It is a chronic disorder of the trigeminal nerve (or 5th cranial nerve). Classic Trigeminal Neuralgia; Spasms of sharp, stabbing pain, often described as like a jolt of lightning The pain is confined to the area served by the branches of the TN nerve: lower jaw, upper jaw, cheek, eye, and forehead. The pain may include one, two or all three branches of the TN nerve. Pain is almost always on one side of the face, most commonly the right-hand side. The pain is usually provoked by a light touch on the face, movements of the face (and therefore of the mouth), touching the side of the nose or even a light breeze. Trigger points are usually around the nose and lip. The pain might disappear by itself for weeks, even months, and then return. Atypical TN Aching, burning pain, mainly in the cheek, upper jaw and sometimes lower jaw. It is less likely to happen in the eye and forehead area. A trigger point is more difficult to define than in classic (typical) TN. Sometimes, after a long period, classic TN can also be accompanied by atypical TN. This leads to a combination of the sharp, electric shock-like pain, plus the dull aching pain.

30 seconds of madness **Doug Fry**

My jaw vibrates,
and pain engulfs my face.

If not the teeth, it's the gums,
but must find the source...

My jaw vibrates, it's so intense,
It's so pernicious.

It's making no sense,
this thirty seconds of madness.

My Jaw Condition is my Alarm Clock **Doug Fry**

This is a pain condition in the jaw , which has been diagnosed but will only be cured by operation. Meanwhile medication is the finest relief particularly inhalants,which get into the main facial organs.

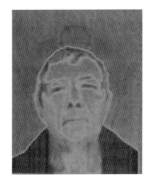

Sometimes I have some very low moments. For instance the pain becomes unbearable when it travels up the facial nerve to the eye. I then get very confused as to The medication that best suits my degree of pain as it could be a sinus problem, or a bout of trigeminal neuralgia.

Doug's artwork
Above:
Self portrait

In fact, another low point is when extreme seasonal conditions affect my jaw and prevent my partaking in exhibitions, as I find it hard getting a body of work together. This is very much unlike me but has a major influence on my art progress. I have always maintained that my condition is as much about relief as the very pain itself. My pain could be identified as intermittent but I openly admire, those unlike myself, who are victims of constant pain.

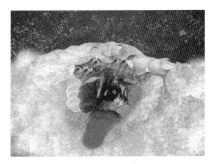

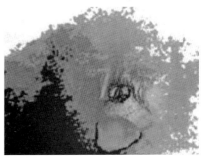

Of the few pieces of advice I could possibly offer one would be to immerse oneself into activities to take the mind off one's condition and maintain a positive approach throughout.

Gordian Bailey uses a wheelchair, powered by himself! He writes, paints and reads with passion. Gordian lost his beloved wife in 2003.

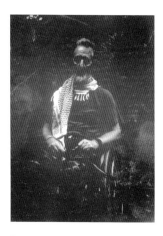

Pinhole
photograph of
Gordian by
David Wise, in
the garden at
Sunlight
in July 2009.

Fist of my heart
Gordian Bailey

The fist in my heart
Red vein of of that thought
The twist in my heart
The death of my wife!

The fury of my faith
Destroyed in a gasp
Jesus be damned!
We prayed through the fight.

The fist in my heart forever
Forever clenched tight.
I am a lucky man
No need to do it again
I have a fist now and not just a heart.

Fortress Fugitive
Gordian Bailey

Higher than the man
The wall divides
Added protection, spiked
To repel, old and established.

The guardian outside the wall
Hears the cries of solitude
From the trapped
And waits to protect

To escape is easy
To make the decision
Is not

For me, the partnerships that people create seem to help us cope with our illness; which becomes part of the partnership.

Marriage **Tina Lawlor Mottram**
(read from left to right as usual!)

The implied.
The absent.
The always.
The straightforwardly direct.
The saving grace.
No penalities.
And the third.

- The present.
- The imperceptible.
- The lack.
- The opposite.
- The great mistake.
- The second chance.
- Etcetera.

Charlie has written many poems throughout his life and this project. This is one he selected for publication.

Flower
Charlie Wolf

Oh flower that came from the East
Do not fall to the Western beast
And its life of little value
But have for yourself a life that's true.

As you age you will lose petals one by one:
A massive change you will have undergone.
You are in my thoughts hour by hour
For you have brightened my life from sour.

You are of mixed blood and that may be
Because like me you have a destiny:
A destiny that with your brother will unfold
And in the future of stories told.

Your beauty is deep inside and rare
Because like me you really care
For people for whom everything is lost
And have to really count the cost.

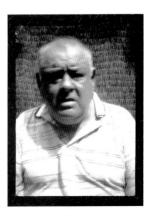

Pinhole photograph of Charlie by David Wise, in the garden at Sunlight in July 2009.

175

Mourning the loss of a loved one is part of the experience of life but that does not make it any less painful. Many other people in the group have lost children and Gill lost her mother, as a result of her own birth. Here are a few of the poems written as a result.

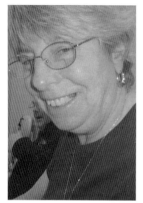

That time of year
Win Gibbons

It's that time of the year again.
That time when it all comes flooding
back to me.

That time when all I wanted to do
is to curl up and die
and follow you into some quiet place.

That time when I wanted to
mop your fevered brow and
whisper sweet lullabies like I did
when you were my baby.

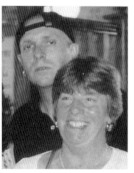

That time when your life on earth
was short and all I would
have is memories of you, my sweet boy
That time of the year comes every year
and with it comes the
joy of once being your Mother.

Top:
Win Gibbons 2010
Below:
Dave and Win 1995

That first time when I held you
to my breast and marvelled in your
Sweetness.

That last time when I heard you
take your last breath and angered
at your passing.

It's that time of the year again.

For the love of a mother, Kit, and my daughter Kate
Gill Solly

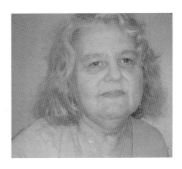

My dearest mother, Kit was her name
Who died at my birth, so I never knew
That special first kiss.
No tender hug did I share from you.
No motherly love; that special bond a mother
and daughter share.
That tender care
was never meant for us.
Not on this Earth, not for me
Never was, never meant to be.

No party dresses, no shopping trips
No sharing bedroom stories and
No you to be a grandma,
as my three grew up.
The ache in my heart will never die
It's here with me, both day and night
No mummy's love, not here for me
Not on this Earth, not for me
Never was, never meant to be.

And then came joy, a daughter for me
I lost her too. Kate, her name was to be.
She didn't live, not on this Earth, not for me.

No pretty ribbons in your hair,
No bedtime stories for us to share
No girly chats, no birthday cakes
no first gentle kiss
No first hug from me to you
I loved you then and I love you still
Not on this earth, not for me
Never was, never meant to be.

I think of you both constantly
Both night and day
Always have and always will.
(continued overleaf)

As long as I live,
with my three beautiful sons
They bring a gift from God
with such love
Then, one day when
the Lord calls me home
Grown old, to that Heaven above

On angels' wings,
you'll wait there for me.
Both Kit the mother I so love
and my daughter Kate,
as a beautiful babe
We will share that
first special hug and kiss

Together for eternity,
we will all share
The love of two mothers,
two daughters
Both Kit and Kate and me.

But for now, life carries on,
as it always does
My heart still aches,
as it always has
I'll love you always,
We'll be there all three.

But not on this Earth,
never was, never meant to be
Not on this Earth, not for me.

A Tree of Light & A Tree of Life **Gill Solly**

A tree of life and a tree of light,
Grows from a seed planted in the ground,
Fed to grow by rain and sun,
Sent from heaven,To nourish and cherish,
Will grow strong with it's branches high above,
The trunk is strong to keep it up,
Roots below that ensure it's future,

Family trees, with their seasons of life,
From Spring to Autumn so we grow,
Spring our beginning with tender blossoms,
As it's cherished and nurtured from mother's arms,
Into our adult life the summer comes,
To meet new love ones, and expand our family,
New lives, marriage and joy for us,
With babies to bring into this world, to cherish and love,
A new generation begins from us has we move into autumn,
And the colours of gold,
Beautiful colours to show our life's fruit,
Friends and loved ones we've met through the years,
Sorrow and joy we've shared with them all,
Then comes winter, joy of grandchildren,
The next generation of the family tree,
For us to cherish and love you see.

As we look back at our family tree and the seasons of life,
We look at the branches above,
Reach into heaven of loved ones past,
With their memories of life once know,
And memory a name sits on those branches dear,
Tender branches below, so sweet and so small,
Blossoming for the future, who and whatever it calls,
Down to the strong trunk, at the centre of our lives,
That gives us such hope at such difficult times,
So full of strength, faith, hope and love,
And healing for us,
Then to the roots that grow in the grounds,
Feeding the future so that the family tree,
So that names can go on, and we're never gone,

Long after we have flourished and flown,
So the point of the family tree is simple you see,
The light is the faith and the healing we need
To get us through pain and illness, sadness and loss
But also comes love that is sent from above,
Which gives us joy and comfort through life.
So you see all three of these are needed
Faith, hope and love.
But the most important is love,
Sent from God from above.

Ken Hopper

Ken is an artist. His paintings can be seen in the colour section of this book. During the project, Ken got psoriasis, which he describes in this piece.

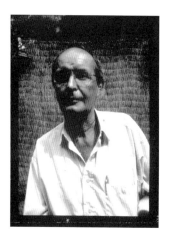

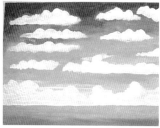

Psoriasis

Debilitating -
invasion of my body -
I am not free from this
or ever shall be -
I realise that I should have
more control over my mind -
My thoughts -
That I am inflicting this upon myself -
I should be stronger in
my actions of what I want -
Of what I should achieve -
Is the same weakness still there? -
The hour is getting late -
If not now, then when?
Has it always been when?
Have I written myself off?
I can't do that -
That would be death.

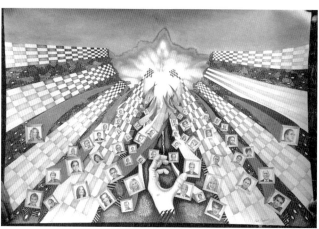

Ken made a conscious link with the condition and later wrote 'You made me aware of my physical self interfering with my mind. It is an ongoing process'

Ken's paintings are in the colour section

James Solly

James is the computer expert in his family, who has kept Gill and Derrick linked with the group by email and also by helping to update the group website with details of their support group for Cerebellar Ataxia. James also designed the cover for this book - his colour sketch can be seen in the colour section.

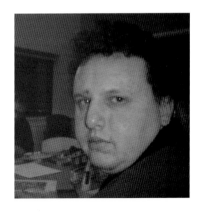

His beautiful tree paintings, seafronts and other artwork are shown below, throughout the book and also in the colour section.

A man of few words, James has happily painted his way through our creative project. These paintings can be seen in the colour section.

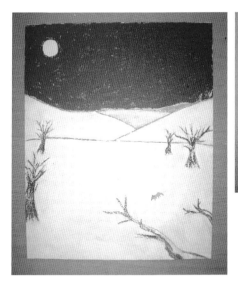

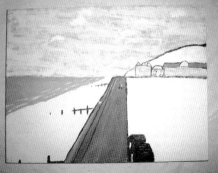

Tania

It's been a while, exhausted now
High hopes bring wasted fear
I wonder if I'll repeat these words
Alone, this time, next year...

People, places, worn out faces,
Dreams that can't be hidden
I disappeared, you walked away
Some things, you know can't be forgiven...

Sadness, regret, self pity, injustice
Darkened bricks all sat on my shoulder
Wonderful memories of a past and a future
But hey, I'm so glad I got older...

So I'll dream of life and all that she sings
No more tears, nor pain, nor grief
Just Magical skies and sweet fireflies
And a world full of warm self belief...

Tania's
artwork can be
seen in the
colour section.

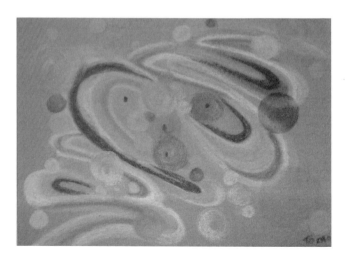

Cathy Sutton

Like most people who took part creating artwork, Cathy said prior to starting that she couldn't do it. 'I never knew I was artistic. Look! I've made a collage' with a wide grin. I like to think that it is *that* smiling feeling that I captured in this photo of Cathy taken at a local park, called Hillyfields.

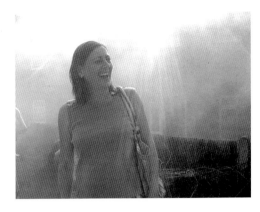

Collage is so easy because you can work with printed images and words and recreate them to become your idea. The one (right) which Cathy created, says 'Say No to Kingsnorth' refers to plans to build a new coal powered station at Kingsnorth, visible from close to the Sunlight centre and a hot issue locally.

Cathy got involved in the project as a local councillor. She's attended very regularly and says 'This is such a worthwhile project.' She's also very kindly decided to donate some of her ward funds to allow the project to contine, after our lottery funding finishes.

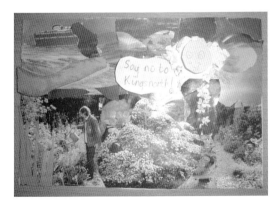

Tina Lawlor Mottram

For me, this whole project has been involved in slowing down time while in meditation, finding time to create and also time to deliberate on our illnesses in ways not medical and logical. I wanted to look at the nature of time itself. Coupled with the tree theme, which I've been playing with for years, these poems are a summary of the year 2009-2010 for me.

Khronos: In Greek = time. In English 'chrono-' = relating to time.
Time as we ordinarily think of it.Fleeting time with birth and death. Clock time.
Kairos: In Greek = opportunity.
Birth and death may be illusions. It's possible to be in more than one place at a time. Time travel. No beginnings and no endings?

Increate Tina Lawlor Mottram

To render capable and suitable
to accept the increate
to qualify its creation with
the dial of a mariner's compass
to play a leading card in the game of
chance, drizzle and abundance.

To connect, to unite, to join
both khronos and kairos as
forces in space and time.

Projecting the germ of seed outwards,
towards a changing yet time-still maturity
leaving to one side the ingrate.

The wonder-working, mirific abundance
of the timeless
the meeting of this and that
the juncture of the increate
the meeting of the beneficent and
the latent:
A potent mix!

Freedom Tree **Tina Lawlor Mottram**

freedom is relative
top and bottom of the pile
river deep, mountain high
MPs expenses, Gurkhas' freedoms
the rich get richer; the poor get louder
as it all piles skyscraper high:
the rubbish, the eco mess
the lack of Copenhagen redress
the debt of the poor,
the rich men's pensions.
the fat cats slither
deep undergound
shame! and our thoughts
fly skyward
intrepid
dreams
daring to
float ideas
of possibles
in a world of
more than
inequalities.
DIY with
the what
you believe
in, as
opposed to
gripe with
the what
you do not.
change what
is impossible
dream it. envision it. seed it well.
from little acorns, oak trees grow
educate for ideas
as above, so below

The Tree of Light **Tina Lawlor Mottram**

Breathe in love, fill your body full
Exhale the unnecessary, let it fall
Breathe in love, fill your heart
Exhale, let go anthing that is disturbing you
Feel your feet heavy on the ground
Send roots down, deeper, deepest
Breathe in love, feel it in your feet
Sense the sap rising, through ankles, knees
Breathe in love, earth energy, energise your tired parts
Feel earth energy fill you with food
With water, sunshine, warmth

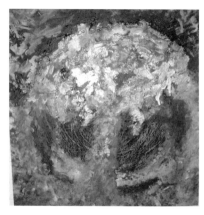

Feel the energy float to your hips,
your abdomen, your back
Breathe in warmth; breathe in precious life
The earth energy rises
Grounds your lower body
You feel securely placed
Above your head, a star; universal love
Connect with it, feel it above your sky
A shower of golden light, winding its way
Feel it fall gently, like
sea mist on your crown
From head to eyes, to throat, to heart
Feel its certain path

Breathe in light, feel it centred in your heart
Breathe in love, mixing with the light
Fill your heart with love and light and earth
Feel your roots grow powerful
Your trunk is strong and wind circled
Your arms feel heavenly, sprouting growths
they become shoots, leaves, flowers
Watch as fruit becomes
Breathe love into them; they carry the seeds
You are a tree; feel your power
Connected to heavens and sky
rooted in the earth, breathing love
on all who pass by

A short verse **Pat Cooper**

I write these few words on Valentine's day,
a day that love is supposed to surround us all.
Expressed by flowers and cards and poetry
for the lucky ones.

Some receive these protestations of love,
totally unaware of the existence of the sender of these gifts,
and they are left with a burning curiosity as to who could have
sent the fine words to one such as them.

Others are expecting something on this, the lover's day,
and are deeply woeful when expectations are not fulfilled,
and for them, the day means nothing.

For those whose wishes do come true,
and pretty cards and flowers are displayed for all to see,
life is wonderful.

Not everything in life is as simple as sending a card or
flowers.
It can be a lot of hard work,
and we do not know what life is going to throw at us.
But through friendships made,
and deeper understanding of others when we meet,
we can say, that like the happy recipients on Valentine's day,
perhaps for a short while,
life is wonderful.

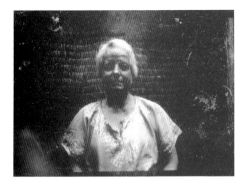

Pinhole
portrait of Pat
in the garden at
Sunlight 2009,
by David Wise

Jonathon Hope

From my own experience, I believe that each and every one of us can overcome our suffering. In most cases, time permitting, that includes overcoming all physical, mental, emotional and spiritual dis-ease that is the root cause of suffering. However, when we have such profound, long lasting and traumatic illnesses as with a long term condition, it takes time, it requires us to take full responsibility for ourselves and for our health. It takes commitment, self exploration, self development and will power. Above all, it takes an open mind, a mind that respects the power of logic, science and medicine, but is not imprisoned by it and hence is also prepared to try out and experiment with other treatment options that deliver healing. By healing I mean returning one to good health with a complete and total sense of well being. To put it another way, true inner and outer healing delivers a reconnection with the joy, excitement, peace and lightness of being that is our birthright.

There are just five steps we can each take to escape and overcome our suffering and ultimately to heal ourselves. Each journey of healing will be different and no two people heal themselves in exactly the same way.

• First, we must resist or overcome the inclination to cut ourselves off from the world, or accept a survival mode mentality, no matter how attractive that coping tactic appears at times. It is vital that we get back into the flow of life. This initial step is mostly about sheer will power and determination i.e. having the strength, despite the pain, the distress, the symptoms, to reconnect with the outside world.

• Second, we need to tackle the physical symptom burden of our disease, by the use of conventional and complementary medicine. In my experience, complementary medicine is more powerful at effectively treating such symptoms than conventional medicine. Without achieving some sense of physical comfort, it is difficult to move onto the next step.

• Third, we can't change our state of health without changing ourself. We must make a conscious decision to change. This is the most important step. No matter how much we are in pain, I know from my own experience that we can leave this suffering behind if we choose. We can get better. It is a great idea to ask for help in doing this. Ask whoever you like. Those around you or your loved ones. Ask the Universe, God, Zero Point Energy, All That Is. Ask the small bird that you notice outside in the snow. Just ask.

• Fourth, we need to start working with our mind to find the key that keeps us inadvertently locked mentally in the prison of our illness or disease. Suffering is an attitude of the mind, not of the body and not of the inner self. Hence we work with the mind and the inner self, through a range of techniques such as meditation, visualisation and affirmations to change our attitudes and release our suffering mindset.

• Fifth, we need to pinpoint the true reason for our illness, our dis-ease. I am not talking about the scientific or medical reason, but the spiritual reason for our illness. Once this is discovered, the final stage of the healing process can begin.

It takes time and it is hard work. But through these five steps, no matter how unimaginable it may be to us, we can achieve good health, discover that there is true, profound meaning in illness and learn to reconnect with our true joyous, light-hearted, light-footed self.

Index 1: Bibliography

Many of these books are available to borrow (for members) from the College of Psychic Studies Library (listed CPS in this Index). Others are available on Amazon, from the British Library and if you're lucky, from secondhand bookshops and friends' libraries...

A Mere Grain of Sand, Ray & Gillian Brown, with Paul Dickson; Tagman Press. 2004.
Studies in Spiritual Healing, A Graham Ikin, The World Fellowship Press Ltd, London. CPS.
Healers and healing, Roy Stemman. Judy Piatkus Publishers Ltd, 1999. CPS.
How to read the aura, W E Butler. Aquarian Press. 1971. CPS.
The Blue Island, William Thomas Stead, Pardoe Woodman, Estelle Stead. Rider & Co.1922.
Spiritual Healing, Daniel J Benor. Vision Publications. 2002. 4 volumes.
The Awakened Mind, Maxwell Cade and Nona Coxhead, Wildwood House Ltd. CPS .
Miracles of healing, Brad Steiger, SH Steiger. Adams Media.com
The seven levels of healing, Lilla Bek and Philippa Pullar. Century Hutchinson Ltd. CPS.
Why people don't heal and how they can, Caroline Myss. Bantam Books. 1998 CPS.
Powers of Healing, Ed Sue Joiner. Time Life Books. 1989.
The teachings of Don Juan, Carlos Castaneda. Penguin. 1970.
The NHS Healer, Angie Buxton-King, Virgin Books, 2004.
My life with Diabetes, Jan de Vries. Mainstream Publishers. 2003.
Living with a long-term illness; Frankie Campling, Michael Sharpe. OUP. 2006
The Power to Heal, David Harvey, Aquarian Press. 1983. CPS.
New Miind, New Body, Barbara B Brown, Hodder & Stoughton, 1974. CPS.
Love, medicine and miracles, Bernie S Siegel, MD, Harper & Row. 1990.
The Aquarian Conspiracy, Marilyn Ferguson. JP Tarcher Inc. ISBN 0-87477-458-6.
The Ancient Maya, Sylvanus G Morley. 1946, SG Morely.
Clairvoyant reality, Laurence LeShan, Turnstone Press Ltd, 1980.
(previously published as The Medium, the mystic and the physicist 1974)
The Therapeutic Touch, Dr Dolores Krieger, Spectrum, 1979.
The Complete Healer, David Furlong. Piatkus, 1995.
The Pocket I Ching; The Richard Wilhelm Translation, Arkana, Penguin Books, 1984.
The Tree of Life, Roger Cook, Avon, 1974.
Extraordinary Encounters, George Chapman, Lang Publishing, 1973, CPS.
Witch Doctor's Apprentice, Nicole Maxwell. 1961, Gollancz, London, 1962.
In Search of Stones, M Scott Peck. Simon & Schuster, 1996.
The Chakras, CW Leadbeater, Quest Books, 1974 (original 1927)
Mysticism, Annie Besant, Theosophical Publishing House, 1914
Spiritualism: A Critical Survey. Edmunds, Simeon. Aquarian Press, 1966.
The Cosmic Serpent, Jeremy Narby. Phoenix. 1995.
Spirit Healing, Harry Edwards, CPS library.
A Guide To The Understanding & Practice Of Spiritual Healing, Harry Edwards.
One Hundred Years of Spiritualism: The Story of the Spiritualist Association of Great Britain, 1872-1912. Roy Stemman, London, 1972.
The Aquarian guide to the new age, Eileen Campbell and JH Brennan, The Aquarian Press, 1990.

• **Cerebellar Ataxia**
National website: www.ataxia.org.uk
• **Kitty's Support Group for Ataxia and Neurological Disorders**
The group meets once a month on Wednesday at St Margaret's and St Peter's church in Rochester, Kent. For more information, contact Gill or Derrick Solly on 01634 813988 or email jamessolly@btinternet.com.
• **Cancer**
www.macmillan.org.uk   Macmillan
• **Living your Life**
Sunlight Development Trust, 105 Richmond Road, ME7 2QA
www.sunlighttrust.org.uk Tel: 01634 338600
• **Online support**
www.healingcancernaturally.com/power-of-thought-to-heal-1.html
www.canceradvice.co.uk/support-groups
• **Temporo Mandibular Joint disorder**
Website: http://forum.tmj.org/
• **Trigeminal Neuralgia**
Website: http://www.tna.org.uk/
Telephone helpline 07786 936120 and email help@tna.org.uk.

College of Psychic Studies
16 Queensberry Place, South Kensington, London SW7 2EB
Tel: 020 7589 3292 Website: http://www.collegeofpsychicstudies.co.uk/
A team of Spiritual Healers, trained at the College, is available for healing at Monday's and Thursday's Healing Clinics, the Group Contact Healing Clinic (three healers with one client) on Wednesdays and also through the weekly Distant Healing Group.

• Monday Healing Clinic Mondays, 11.15am - 4pm (30 minute sessions).
• Wednesday Group Healing Clinic
Clients lie on a couch and three healers work on that one person, bringing down three healing rays simultaneously in a focused way. This is extremely effective for clients who are seriously ill and for those who have already had other forms of healing but still haven't achieved well-being. Wednesdays, 11.15am - 1.30pm (15 minute sessions).
• Thursday Healing Clinic Thursdays 7.15pm - 9.15pm (30 minute sessions).
• Distant healing Group
On Thursday evenings, a group of healers send healing from our sanctuary to those who cannot come for personal healing at the College. Names and details of people requiring this service may be left with Reception during the week.

Ray Brown
To book appointments with Ray Brown and Paul:
Email raybrownenquiries@hotmail.com or telephone 07831 641321.
Website: http://www.raybrownhealing.com
Clinics: Lutterworth, (Leics), Hainault (Essex), Leigh, (Dorking), Bury St
Edmunds, (Suffolk), Chiswell Green, (St Albans) and Brighton. Please get in
touch to book an appointment.

International Church and Healing Fellowship (ICHF)
Head Office, Harmony Country Lodge, Limestone Road,
Burnston, Scarborough YO13 0DG. Website: www.ichf.org.uk
Telephone 01723 871218. Email: admin@ichf.org.uk.

Harry Edwards Healing Sanctuary
Burrows Lea, Hook Lane, Shere, Near Guildford, Surrey, UK GU5 9QG
The Sanctuary at Burrows Lea is the former home of Harry Edwards and he
founded the Charity in 1966. We continue to give contact and distant healing
without charge. Website: http://www.harryedwards.org.uk/
Telephone 01483 202054 or email: healingreception@burrowslea.org.uk

Burrswood Hospital and Place of Healing
Burrswood, Groombridge, Tunbridge Wells, Kent, TN3 9PY
The Dorothy Kerin Trust - a charitable company . Burrswood is a Christian
hospital and place of healing, set in the heart of Kent. Tel: 01892 863687
Website: http://www.burrswood.org.uk

Sue Allen
Website: http://www.sueallentherapies.co.uk/
I am a natural psychic, sensitive, healer, medical intuitive, psychotherapist
and teacher. I specialise in spirit release and psychic attack, clearing
people and places of unwanted energies.

Linda Hinshelwood
Healer at the Wednesday Healing Clinic in the College of PsychicStudies
Website - http:// www.reflexologyandhealing.co.uk

Angie Buxton-King & Graham King
Healers in the NHS at UCLHospital
Website: http://www.angiebuxton-king.com

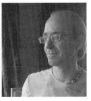

Confederation of Healing Organisations
http://www.confederation-of-healing-organisations.org/
UK Healers http://www.ukhealers.info/

Other Useful sites
Maxwell Cade Foundation
ttp://www.mindmirroreeg.com/w/MaxwellCade.htm
William Thomas Stead resource site:
www.attackingthedevil.co.uk

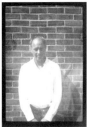

Index 4: Photographers and Picture Credits
• Jonathon Hope
Email: jonathonhope@msn.com
Mobile: 07969 229974

• David Wise
Website: www.davewise.biz
Email: dave@davewise.biz
Mobile: 07864 743157

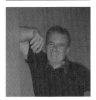

• Derek Wilkinson
Email: Derek.Wilkinson@westking.ac.uk
Mobile: 07984 649777

• Tina Lawlor Mottram
www.serpentinacreations.co.uk / www.serpentinacreations.com
Email: serpentina@blueyonder.co.uk   Mobile: 07966 983935

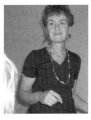

• Cerys Evans
A star photographer and only 7 years old! eg See her work at
number 4 right...

Picture Credits (in order of page appearance)
The author has tried to locate copyright owners for pics and references. Humble
apologies if I have been unable to contact you. Please get in touch and this will be
rectified in any future edition(s).

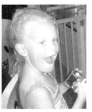

Page no	Many thanks to:
39	Tony Mardel
61	W T Stead Resource Site.
69	Wikipedia
74	Dorothy Kerin, Burrswood Hospital and Place of Healing
78	Rose Gladden; Lindy Cowling, Rose Gladden's grand daughter
80-82	Trustees of the Harry Edwards Healing Sanctuary

Photographers are credited in captions unders pics in the book.
Any other photos were probably snapped by Tina Lawlor Mottram.

Photographers
1. Jonathon Hope
2. David Wise
3. Derek Wilkinson
4. Tina Lawlor
Mottram
5. Cerys Evans

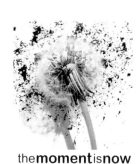

themomentisnow

Themomentisnow!
c/o Sunlight Development Trust
105 Richmond Road, Gillingham, Kent ME7 1LX
01634 338600
www.themomentisnow.org.uk
www.sunlighttrust.org.uk

We are a group of artists, writers and healers working on projects about long term health: expressing the seen and unseen in words and image. We are a constituted community group, working on creative projects linked to

• long term illness; health and healing
• art and environment
• creative writing
• our local community

Our community publisher, themomentisnow! books, can help to get your idea into print. If your project fits within our interest areas, we may be able to provide an ISBN, design and editing services, help with marketing, publicity and sales. For a quote on getting your book published, please get in touch.

For more information, please contact: Tina Lawlor Mottram
01634 319739 / 07966 983935 or serpentina@blueyonder.co.uk

The author

Tina Lawlor was born in Dublin. She studied art at Limerick College of Art and typography to postgraduate level in the then London College of Printing. Her publishing experience was gained at HMSO, Collins Publishers and the Royal Armouries in HM Tower of London, as Design Manager. Homes have included London, Barcelona, Budapest, Prague and Madrid, where she taught a lot of English and learned a few other languages along the way. She's been a correspondent for the Medway Messenger and had lots of poems, stories and art published by Urban Fox Press and Full Circle. She's exhibited artwork at too many shows to list here. Her first volume of poetry 'When the forevers become' was published in 2007. Currently she is the Editor of Sunlight News, a healer in the College of Psychic Studies and also enjoys 3 days as a healer in a school in south London.
She added the Mottram part to her name in 2002 and lives happily with her husband and daughter in Kent.